Praise for *Reiki in Integrative Medicine*

"Lori has been an angel with her passion for helping the frontline healthcare community with Reiki, and they have benefited so much from it."
"Great reading for professionals who care for their own, especially in medical leadership."

Sanjay P. Muttreja, MD, SFHM
Chief of Staff, Southwest Healthcare System

"With compassion and clarity, M. Lori Torok offers a much-needed guide to understanding Reiki and its importance in integrated medicine. Lori's approach is relatable as many of us in the healthcare industry have witnessed and experienced miracles when the mind-body and spirit align. This book offers a guide to understanding Reiki and ways in which we can embrace Reiki to support us in our journey of healing as a provider and a patient."

Manpreet K. Rai, MBA, MA, CRM, LMFT
Reiki Master Teacher

"As a registered nurse, Reiki has brought greater insight into my work and has been an invaluable tool in my personal journey. M. Lori Torok shows how this powerful therapeutic approach, combined with integrative medicine, can bring about deeper levels of healing."

Micaela Larson, BSN, RN, PHN
Reiki II Practitioner

"Lori Torok's *Reiki in Integrative Medicine* provides a concise and evidence-informed overview of Reiki, bridging the gap between complementary therapies and conventional medical practices. It's a helpful resource for both healthcare professionals and patients seeking holistic care."

Heather Norlund, RN

"Lori's brought forth another message we all need to hear: we are 'each responsible for the energies we bring into the world.' This is inclusive in her work and a solid foundation in 'The Forgiveness Project.' *Reiki in Integrative Medicine* is another soul-touching work from Lori—one the world needs and the healing professions of medicine and behavioral health are desperate for."

Mary Scott Carpenter, Owner, CFND Behavioral Health

"I found the book to provide examples of how reiki can assist as a complementary addition to health and healing in the medical realm. Medical Reiki synergistically assists healing without contraindications, providing …overall health and safety and promoting positive outcomes."

Jennifer Duffy, RN, EMT-P

"With its easy-to-understand language, Lori's thoughtful and well-researched second book takes the "woo-woo" out of the wonder that is Reiki and provides a clear path for those curious about the benefits of Reiki and how its integration may offer a deeper, more holistic opportunity for healing."

Jennifer Voss
Reiki Master Teacher

"Lori did an amazing job breaking down the facets of Reiki for ALL to comprehend with this book. It excites and provides me hope for the future of Healthcare. This book is the pebble, initiating a ripple throughout standard medicine, helping us realize the importance not to just sustain life, but to feed the souls of our patients. [This book provides] research and facts into the advantages of incorporating [Reiki] alongside standard medicine. I can't wait to share it with others."

Kimberly Sherwood, RCT

"Reiki in Integrative Medicine is a must-read for anyone interested in learning more about how the beautiful energy of Reiki can enhance their healing journey. Being a Reiki practitioner, I look forward to recommending this simple and easy-to-read book to anyone...curious about how Reiki works to enrich the healing of our body, mind, and spirit."

Michelle Jones
Reiki Master Teacher

Reiki in Integrative Medicine

What Reiki Therapy Is, What it Isn't, and How It Supports Healing

M. LORI TOROK

EIGHTH RAY
PUBLISHING

Published in the United States by

Eighth Ray Publishing

Escondido, CA

www.eighthraypublishing.com

Text © M. Lori Torok, 2025

The moral and energetic rights of the author have been asserted.

The material in this book is used for informational purposes only and not intended to diagnose, treat, or prevent any condition or disease or as a substitute for medical care. Please consult your physician or healthcare specialist regarding the suggestions and recommendations made in this book. Neither the author nor the publisher can be held responsible for any loss, claim, or damage arising from the use or misuse of the suggestions made, the failure to take medical advice, or any material on third-party websites. Additionally, this book does not provide training in the use or practice of Reiki or its attunements; please consult a qualified Reiki Master Teacher.

Cover and Interior Book Design: Jennifer Federico Stimson

ISBN Paperback 979-8-9881057-6-3

ISBN Hardback 979-8-9881057-5-6

ISBN Kindle eBook 979-8-9881057-7-0

ISBN Audio Book 979-8-9881057-8-7

www.ReikiIntegrativeMedicine.com

~ For Raven Keyes ~
The Reiki flame continues to grow.

Table of Contents

CHAPTER 3

Care of the Soul in Clinical Settings 63

CHAPTER 4

Evidence-based Studies of Reiki's Effectiveness................83

CHAPTER 5

Finding a Qualified Reiki Practitioner 91

CHAPTER 6

Talking About Reiki

For most of us, there are key points when we can identify the exact moment when a door was flung open, and we walked through and kept moving forward on a new path. We may even see it replaying in our inner eye's timeline: there was life before the door and life after. These doorways often mark moving homes, changing jobs, starting or ending relationships, or unexpected life changes, like births or deaths. One of these doors brought an element of all these for me—shift, change, birth, and death.

One of the first times I heard the word Reiki spoken was in meditation. I had asked for guidance on healing something in my physical body. I expected to hear/feel that I should eat more kale or drink wheatgrass juice or something along the lines of nutritional healing. Instead, I heard a voice deep within me, but not me, clearly say, *"Learn Reiki."* Having never heard this Japanese word spoken before, I didn't know it was pronounced "ray-key," and I thought, *"Oh, that's how you say that word."*

Speaking with my inner voice, I replied, *"That sounds hard. If I don't do that, what else can I do?"* At that moment, the energy collapsed. My connection was disrupted. I felt the seriousness of the voice guiding me, but I didn't know where to begin. I thought this meant returning to school, and I wasn't entirely sure I wanted to do that. I was already a college professor, chair of two programs, artistic director of a dance company, and, most importantly, the mother of an active five-year-old. Unsure about what to do with the guidance, I moved on with my day and went to work.

Later that day, a colleague from another department knocked at my office door. We were acquaintances and had worked together on a few interdisciplinary projects, but this was the first time he had come to see me. I invited him in, and after a few pleasantries, he shared with me that he was studying Reiki and was at the second level of his training, Reiki II. I asked why he decided to stop by to tell me about this on this particular day, and he said that he was just walking by and had an inner feeling to stop and talk to me about Reiki. I was dumbfounded. I told him about my guidance that morning, and it seemed inevitable that I needed to find a class to begin learning Reiki, and soon.

After some research, I found a teacher offering sessions out of her home who seemed like a good fit and made an appointment. Appreciating the value of scholarship and research, I thought I should first see what Reiki was before attending the first session, and I attempted to read as much as I could about the topic. At that time, however, in 2011, there wasn't much, and what I did find was rather esoteric and vague.

A couple of days later, I experienced my first Reiki session. From what I can recall, it was lovely and relaxing, though not much more. I was rather skeptical of it all and reserved judgment. I felt like I was still researching rather than receiving. I was in no rush, so I circled the trailhead a bit before running down the path. Honoring my angelic guidance, I registered for Reiki I training. By that weekend, I was in a small class of five students, all eager to learn. I soon found that people come to this work for various reasons.

My motivation for being there felt a little ungrounded since it came through inner guidance. Given that my work to that point had been practical and scholarly, I did not share exactly how I found myself in the class. To be honest, I was still a bit skeptical.

After an introductory period in which we were taught about Dr. Usui and the history of Reiki in Japan and its development in the United States and the West, the teacher prepared us for what she called an "attunement." For this, we sat in the teacher's high-back dining room chairs, a few feet away from each other. We were asked to close our eyes and focus inwardly; it is a sacred experience. When the teacher came to me, she moved around my chair, placing her hands on mine and ceremonially moving them into different positions, doing some breathwork, and placing her hands on my shoulders.

I felt an inner jolt, as I realized that this was the same as a recurring dream I had been having for months. In my dream, I was sitting in a high-backed wooden chair, and an older woman, a grandmother figure (but no one I knew), was moving around me in some sort of ceremony, placing her hands on me and doing some sort of breathy chant.

I would usually wake up at this point, wondering, *"What is the meaning of this dream?"* But at that moment, during the first attunement for Reiki I, I knew, without a doubt, that I was exactly where I was supposed to be—that I had been truly guided to this work. Everything in my life had conspired to bring me to this moment in time. This was the door I was meant to walk through.

The Calling

I completed my training class (the first of three), learned some specialized work with Reiki, and began using its healing energies on myself and sharing it with family and friends. Eventually, my friends' friends started to request sessions. A de facto practice was developing without that being my intention. Not having an extra room in our home, my husband and I turned our dining room into a treatment room, and he and my daughter would leave the house so I could give sessions. This was a time of great transformation for my family, led by the beautiful healing energies of Reiki, and I was grateful for my husband's support. Moreover, Reiki had become such a welcomed practice in my life that I began to secretly long to spend more time working with Reiki rather than heading off to work to sit behind a desk.

For a couple of years, Reiki was a tremendous presence in the family household, and we all benefitted from its loving presence. Then, one day while teaching a dance class, I ruptured my calf muscle. It was a severe injury and kept me from bearing weight on that leg for an extended period. Even after two months, with my Reiki and all the doctor's care and physical therapy, my calf was seemingly not healing, and I finished the semester on crutches. I changed doctors for a second opinion and sought all sorts of assistance—prayer, meditation, and Reiki, but was still no wiser as to why this injury was not healing, and in fact, not getting better at all.

Increasingly, I was asking for higher guidance as to the deeper meaning behind this injury because I had been healthy at the time. *"What was really going on here?"* At the same time, and in no part *because* of the injury, my job was becoming more stressful and less joyful. Managing program reviews, curriculum rewrites, scheduling templates, and district reports had taken over my daily schedule far more than teaching. These administrative stresses had long been making me wish for change, and I was still too far from retirement to linger in an unhappy situation.

After several weeks of discussion with my husband, we agreed that it was time for me to leave the job that had been home for fourteen years. I knew Reiki was going to be a part of my future, but I did not know exactly how or what that would look like. Composing a letter of resignation was not an easy task, but it was the right door to go through. When I completed the letter and sent it, I pushed my chair away from the desk and stood up without an ounce of pain! For the first time in months, I was completely pain-free. I was in a state of disbelief. How could this be? What just happened? I was walking with no pain, not even a residual stiffness. Nothing. It was completely healed. This immediately confirmed that this was the right door, even if I did not yet know what was on the other side.

A few weeks later, the final day at work arrived, and it was time to clear out my office. I received a call from the Vice President of Instruction asking to meet with me. I was a bit apprehensive and had inwardly decided that I would not be sharing anything about Reiki with my superiors, as they just would not understand, and I did not want to be considered some kook who was going off to do woo-woo work, after so many years of respectable scholarship and teaching.

When I arrived, the VP was waiting for me, and we sat down to talk. He said that he wanted to make sure that I was okay because "people don't usually leave these sorts of jobs." He wanted to know what my plans were for the future. I took a deep breath and told him that I had been doing Reiki energy work for the past two years and that it had been an extraordinary journey of growth and healing. I paused and then told him that I was following deep inner guidance to do this work full-time. There were a couple of moments of silence. I expected perhaps an eyeroll or a chuckle. But it never came.

Instead, the VP shared his spiritual journey and how important that has been for him. He let down his usual guarded demeanor, and I saw the light in his eyes. He leaned in and said he completely understood, "This is a calling! You are following a calling!" He said that he was relieved and knew that I would be okay and that I would be taken care of by the one who had called me. We then spoke a little more about Reiki and other business matters, and he reminded me to see HR before I officially left the college. It just so happens that I already had an appointment for later that day.

I left the meeting extremely surprised, pleasantly so. However, I was disappointed in myself. I had expected someone with the VP's title, credentials, and formality to disregard or dismiss my work with Reiki. But that was all me. That was my bias, not his. I heard a deep call from my soul to never again disrespect others regarding sharing about Reiki. I had heard that people do or would understand this work. Everyone has had spiritual or mystical experiences that they cannot explain in any other way. I knew I must trust that this work was very much needed, and to be led to those whom I could help with Reiki. So, I went on to my appointment with HR, now committed to truth and trust, while I prayed for the right words.

The head of HR took me into a private room and asked a few questions to satisfy the exit interview and to fill out all the paperwork. She then asked the question, "So what will you be doing?" I took a deep breath and began to tell her about Reiki. It wasn't long before I mentioned working with beautiful angelic guides who had led me to this path. She had tears in her eyes and said, "I need this. When can I make an appointment?" I was taken by surprise and thought maybe she was being polite. However, she went on to tell me that that very morning she was asking for assistance from above, she was asking for a sign, and now she is having this conversation with me. She took this as her sign.

If I had not learned the lesson earlier from the VP to trust, share, and know that people truly need this, then I am not sure the HR conversation would have happened. She made an appointment and visited my home office several times over the next few months to receive Reiki, and I trust she received everything she needed. She left her job at the college not long after I did.

From that moment on, standing in the doorway of change, I learned a most important lesson. Reiki is relevant, and it is very much needed. The hour is late, and there is no time to sit back and hope that people will respect what you do. I am not waiting for permission to be who I am meant to be.

I hear fairly regularly from Reiki clients and students alike that they don't speak to others about this work. They are certain their family, friends, or colleagues wouldn't understand. Doctors, nurses, first responders, professional athletes, churchgoers, teachers, those in government service, and so many others think they need to keep Reiki quiet because other people just wouldn't understand. One sector, in particular, is quietly seeking the relaxation and healing of Reiki but is fearful of ever speaking about it. God bless the people of our military. If they only knew that the US government's Office of Veteran's Affairs (VA) recognizes Reiki as one of the "Complementary and Integrative Approaches in the VA." We will discuss more about this later.

Care for the Caregiver

A few months ago, I was invited to speak at a symposium for the Southwest Healthcare System, which included our three local community hospitals in the Inland Empire of Southern California. This was a dinner for those doctors, nurses, hospital personnel, board members, and community members interested in providing a better environment for hospital workers. The overarching theme of the talks that evening was about the health and culture within the hospital. This was a "Culture of Safety Event presented by Med Staff." They were honoring and celebrating the work of Dr. Timothy McDonald and his nationally recognized Beta HEART program, which supports open, honest communication within the hospital hierarchy to better care for the doctors and nurses who experience secondary trauma as part of their daily work.

My part of the program was called "Care for the Caregiver" and was intended to introduce healthcare workers to Reiki and its benefits in body, mind, and spirit healing.

Knowing that my audience was filled with science-based healthcare workers, I prepared a presentation focused almost entirely on data-driven studies and evidence-based materials that would be a dispassionate delivery of charts, graphs, and numbers. I get it, this is a world that needs quantified proof. I thought I was meeting them where they were, on their terms. And I am glad that was my approach; in a way, it was exactly what was needed.

However, that was not the tone of the other speakers. They spoke of the need for love, compassion, understanding, and care. They spoke of the heart of healthcare and the need for doctors and nurses to live authentically and be able to speak honestly. Most impressively, Dr. Timothy McDonald talked about the willingness to apologize when something goes wrong, and when mistakes are made, and he graciously spoke of the value of Reiki in clearing heavy energies and helping to heal in difficult times. He stood at the podium, praising the work of Reiki and its value to the hospital community.

Once again, I found myself staring into the face of a higher truth. The bias was mine, not theirs. I was ready to be dismissed or even ridiculed, or, in the best-case scenario, simply tolerated, and yet I was welcomed—Reiki was welcomed. The group in attendance asked questions that went far beyond the charts and graphs I provided. They wanted to know more about the *heart* of the healing, the *soul* of Reiki, and how it could assist their patients.

After my talk, I was approached by at least a dozen people who wanted to talk about their experiences with energies that they could not explain, their need for the work of Reiki, and how they wanted to offer Reiki to their staff, their students, and their patients. One, a Marine from a local base, spoke to me about wanting to make Reiki more readily available for those suffering from post-traumatic stress disorder (PTSD).

Throughout the next year, I periodically offered free monthly "Reiki Experiences" to everyone in attendance, including all medical personnel and first responders. These Saturday sessions were given by my Reiki Master graduates and myself at my Reiki Center. Doctors came in before their rounds or after a long night shift, therapists stopped in on their days off, and first responders and their spouses came to these free thirty-minute sessions to experience Reiki firsthand. The experiences were outstanding. Many sent their family in for full sessions, and a few even began learning Reiki themselves.

What I realized, though, is that there needed to be a book that describes Reiki for those who are interested but perhaps have not yet experienced this form of healing. And Reiki is not something you want to learn from random internet videos or social media posts. I also appreciate that you may feel a little skeptical too. I get it. I was right there. I, too, did not trust the responses of others. But that was me; my bias, not theirs. I know now that Reiki meets the individual where they are. It is time we trust that, by talking about Reiki from a place of knowledge and firsthand experience. It is time to replace worn-out personal biases and assumptions about things we do not understand with lived experience, scientific research, and an openness to change.

That is why this book was written. It is for anyone interested in the truth about Reiki—to discover first-hand experiences and facts about what Reiki is, what it is not, and how it can support your healing journey. This book includes the latest information at the time of publication, and I invite you to visit www.ReikiIntegrativeMedicine.com for updates.

CHAPTER 1
What Is Reiki?

Reiki is a Japanese word for "universal life energy" or "spiritual life force." "Rei" means mysterious, spirit, or universal, and "ki" is the life energy or animating force flowing through all living things (in Chinese, this is known as *chi* or *qi*). Reiki is a non-invasive relaxation technique that utilizes the flow of *ki/chi* to return the body, mind, and spirit to its natural integrated state of health and well-being.

Reiki, being the life force, flows through all living things and can be accessed as a personal tool for healing. With some training and receiving the Reiki attunements, you can self-administer Reiki, empowering yourself to maintain your health and balance. Reiki may also be given by a Reiki practitioner—one who has undergone a series of attunements, training, and an extended period of transformative self-healing so they can effectively transmit this energy to others. The professional practitioner has attained what is known as Reiki III training and may be designated as a Reiki Practitioner, Reiki Master, or Reiki Master Teacher.

Although there are dozens of forms of Reiki, what is most commonly known as Reiki in the Western world comes to us through the lineage of its founder, Dr. Mikao Usui. In March 1922, Dr. Usui (known as Usui Sensei in Japan) received Reiki through Divine enlightenment on Mt. Kurama, a sacred mountain located just north of Kyoto, after an intense extended period of meditation and fasting. He learned to use and transmit this energy to others for spiritual growth and physical healing. Dr. Usui went on to create a system to work with this spiritual energy, which he called Reiki, to heal and teach the work to others.

In the early twentieth century, other forms of hands-on energy healing were already being used in Japan, and some of those systems were even called Reiki. However, the roots of the "laying on of hands" for healing go back much further and find their place in sacred texts and ancient belief systems throughout history. It is not as new age as you might think, as it could be argued that Reiki is a return to ancient traditions of self-empowerment, traditional medicine, and our direct personal relationship with the Divine.

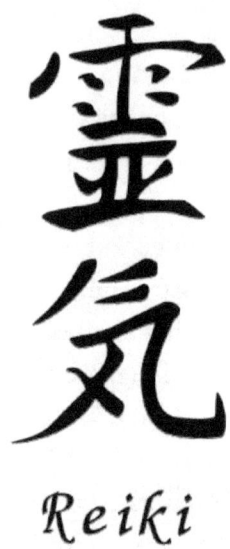

Reiki

Japanese kanji for Reiki (MLTorok/CanvaPro)

Reiki is not a religious belief, and specific beliefs are not required for the recipient or the practitioner. People of any religious beliefs or no belief may find Reiki a supportive practice. Even skeptics find that a Reiki practice, or even a single session, provides relaxation and calm beyond what the mind can create for itself.

Reiki does not need us to believe in it for it to work. However, if someone is determined to fight the flow of Reiki energy, they will likely succeed, as resistance to energy is also energy. Being of a Divine loving nature, Reiki will never force its way and flow where it is unwanted. That is simply the law of free will, which Reiki will always honor. Reiki, being energy, will flow easily through the open door of the one who invited it. It is highest and best to approach Reiki with an open heart and mind. Nothing more is needed.

The Reiki Principles or Reiki Gokai

Dr. Usui taught five simple Reiki principles, or precepts, known in Japanese as *Reiki Gokai* ("go," meaning five; "kai," meaning shell, principle, society) to assist practitioners, recipients, and students on their Reiki paths. These are not about the words themselves or beliefs in the words, but they are spiritual affirmations that support greater health and vitality and invite happiness through an uplifted mindset:

> *Just for today, do not anger or worry.*
>
> *Just for today, be humble.*
>
> *Today, I will count my many blessings.*
>
> *Today, I will do my work honestly.*
>
> *Today, I will be kind to every living creature.*
>
> **The Reiki Gokai, Dr Usui**

We can practice this uplifted mindset and bring the principles of Reiki into our daily lives by being more mindful of our energetic intention:

Living Just for Today

This is a beautiful understanding that we are beings of limitations. We can only take one day, one moment, at a time. This statement, repeated throughout the principles, reminds us of our presence, here and now, for all healing takes place in the now. This acknowledges the mental discipline necessary for the work of Reiki. Dr. Usui reminds us that we control only this moment, or in this case, today.

Be Aware of Anger

Anger is one of the lowest vibrations on the planet and the opposite of the loving, healing energies of Reiki. Anger reminds us that we are over-concerned with things we cannot control and is closely related to disappointment and frustration. Detachment is the key to being an observer of the world, without letting the *dis*-ease of anger take hold of the soul. To attempt to let go of all anger may be overwhelming. However, Dr. Usui asks that we commit to being anger-free, just for today. Tomorrow will take care of itself.

Let Go of Worry

If we are not in the true presence of living in the moment, just for today, the mind may have us falsely believe that we are in control of tomorrow. Over-concern for the future shows up as worry, anxiety, or stress. Come back to today, this moment, here and now. Release the projections of tomorrow, and worry is vanquished. Just for today, do not worry. Tomorrow, we can commit again if we so choose, but that is not the work of today.

Live with Humility

Reiki flows through a clear channel when we are attuned to receive it. This channel must resonate with the highest and best vibrational qualities. The channel is not arrogant or boastful in any way but humble in spirit and recognizes the true honor of holding the healing essence of unconditional love and infinite light. The Reiki practitioner, the channel of Reiki, is in service to this light and must remain humble for its purity.

Remember Gratitude

Gratitude opens the door to the healing power of Reiki, and for that purpose, Dr. Usui reminds us to count our many blessings. In remembering the blessings that life gives to us, we expand our life force in a higher connection to all that is good. Reiki energy has an uplifting, effervescent quality, and the one receiving its blessings or channelling it for the good of others must have an uplifted countenance. The law of vibration explains this principle: Like vibrates like. Energy vibrates sympathetically and requires that those seeking the higher vibrational octaves also resonate with a heightened energetic frequency. Gratitude is one of the keys that assists us in raising our vibration. Remember the good; recall the blessings of life, and we become a channel of the greater good.

Working in Service

There are a couple of differing translations of this line in the original Usui Sensei Gokai. One states, "Today, I will do my work with integrity;" another states, "I will do the work I am meant to do." They both describe a similar quality, which is authenticity. In Reiki, there is no falseness—no one is trying to sell us anything or offering anything that is not truthful. The authentic Reiki practitioner is in service to the Light of Reiki, not their own ego or personal gain, nor is the practitioner trying to prove anything. In this, there is great honor in the work, knowing that Reiki's healing light is not for financial or personal wealth but serves on a much higher octave beyond material accounts. Reiki is deeply spiritual work.

Demonstrating Kindness to All

The final precept of Reiki asks us to treat all living creatures with kindness. Noting that this goes beyond human beings to all living creatures, we include the animal kingdom, plant kingdom, mineral kingdom, and perhaps beings of the spiritual kingdom. This kindness is compassion—an open gentleness of spirit—that expands our hearts and minds to feel the oneness of all in great honor. There is a deeper implication in this final principle: that kindness must also include the self, for we, too, deserve the same loving care that we extend to all living creatures. In the compassionate light of Reiki, we are one.

Where Does Reiki Energy Come From?

Reiki is life force energy that comes from the source of life, the Divine Creator, Mother-Father God, if you will. The core understanding is that we, as humans, did not create ourselves; we did not create our souls. We came from somewhere else, and the energetic imprint from the Creator/Source still flows through us. It is a pure and loving energy beyond anything known or created by humans.

The practitioner does not *do* the healing but is the conduit, channel, or bridge for this high-vibrational energy. Reiki—being Source energy—does the healing; the practitioner is the channel of the healing energy. However, Reiki differs from other biofield energy healing and is described most succinctly in this way:

> *The Reiki practitioner, unlike with other energy-healing modalities, becomes a channel, a conduit, for the healing energies of Divine Light and Love to flow through the practitioner to the one receiving the healing, whether it is mineral, plant, animal, or human. Unlimited in potential, Reiki can do no harm, as the intention is Light and Love. Reiki can heal anything and everything.*[1]

It is a tremendous gift, an honor, to become a channel of Divine Light and Love, and it carries a responsibility. The Reiki practitioner must be dedicated to a path of purification to hold the sacred light. The Reiki practitioner does not need to be perfect—hardly. However, there are great rewards for those who strive to dedicate themselves to a path of physical, mental, emotional, and spiritual upliftment. Reiki itself may assist us in letting go of the very habits and lower vibrational choices we are ready to release. Setting an intention to heal unwanted dysfunctions and patterns is an effective and rewarding personal use of Reiki.

The Difference Between Healing and Curing

Whether Reiki is self-administered or given through a qualified practitioner, Reiki is a healing practice. When we step into the energies of Reiki, healing will always take place. However, it is important to understand that there is a difference between healing and curing. Within the healing practice of Reiki, the blessing of a cure may also unfold; however, with Reiki, the goal is a deeper level of healing, which includes body, mind, and spirit.

Being life force energy, Reiki will always raise the vibration of the one receiving its energies. It can be no other way: the higher lifts the lower. We now understand that it is called "entrainment," whereby living systems oscillate and integrate with their environments. The frequency that is higher and, thus, stronger will energetically lift the vibration of the lower. Physics and the fields of biomagnetism and magnetocardiography demonstrate this principle in the heart's electromagnetic field, which has been proven to be a stronger and higher oscillator than the brain's electromagnetic field. Thus, where and how the heart resonates, the organs and glands of the rest of the body will follow, head to toe—and, perhaps, outward into the subtle energy bodies or the surrounding biofield, as well.

That being said, medicine in the Western world is racing toward cures—seeking to eliminate diseases, to be symptom-free. That is completely understandable, as we have set ourselves up to be in battle with the disease rather than to be in alignment with health. We fight cancer and are at war with infectious diseases of all sorts. We are set up for the fight, but are we preparing the way for health?

Integrative medicine, Reiki specifically, holds space for light, health, vitality, and (dare I say) love, for it is these that flow with health. Energetically speaking, how can we be at peace unless we call in the higher vibrations of love as part of our healing? Reiki is love, and it is love that heals.

Miraculous cures have taken place with Reiki; they happen every day. The Reiki practitioner will hold space for the miracle with every session. However, that is not the only measure of health, nor is it the practitioner's goal. The Reiki practitioner holds space of Divine light and love—unconditional love and infinite light, blessings of the Divine presence. In alignment with the Divine plan, Reiki can heal anything and everything, as it has unlimited potential.

Reiki is not sought for the promise of a cure for a particular disease. Reiki is sought to bring strength and light, and in that, great relaxation and comfort may be found—ease within the *dis*-ease. Healing is often likened to the layers of an onion, and there are many causes, layers, to the dysfunctional patterns or disruptive energies that surround and bring density to someone's energetic life, the biofield. Reiki will always be helpful in these matters. Reiki will always bring healing, and on occasion, it accompanies the cure.

Understanding how energy and healing work, can you see how Reiki can benefit those undergoing medical treatments?

Reiki and Medicine

Reiki is not a form of medicine in the Western physical sense, but it is considered integrative, complementary, or collaborative medicine in the metaphysical sense. Whereas medical doctors and nurses tend to our health on the molecular-chemical and psycho-physical planes, Reiki addresses healing at the metaphysical or the soul level. What a powerful combination, indeed, when someone feels cared for on all levels of their being.

It is important to state that Reiki practitioners are not doctors or nurses (although many in these fields are also practitioners, and the number is growing). Reiki practitioners do not diagnose, treat, or prescribe medicine. Reiki practitioners work at different levels of the human experience, the metaphysical experience of vibrational frequency and the healing potential of unconditional love. This is also why so many medical professionals find themselves called to learn Reiki, to return to that deep inner calling as healers within their chosen fields, beyond insurance companies, paperwork, and the limitations of the hospital hierarchies.

More than sixty US hospitals in America have adopted Reiki as a regular part of patient services. According to the Institute for Integrative Healthcare, more than a thousand Reiki programs are operating in US hospitals. Still, these numbers are always changing, so it is hard to know exactly how many informal Reiki programs are running in our hospitals, sometimes housed in the spiritual care wing of a medical facility. We will discuss this topic in more detail in Chapter 3, Integrative Medicine, Medical Reiki, and Clinical Settings.

Who Uses Reiki?

Reiki is used, both regularly and intermittently, by people of all ages and stages of life who lead ordinary 21st-century lives to relieve stress, overcome difficult situations, deal with pressures of work or personal life stressors, help eliminate pain at the physical, mental, and emotional levels, help deal with PTSD and past traumatic experiences, relieving heavy emotions like grief, fear, anger, anxiety, or navigating life's challenges and changes.

Many forms of Reiki are flourishing worldwide, as people from all walks of life, belief systems, and career paths are learning how to use it for their health and vitality. Once you understand the foundations of Reiki, a Reiki I training class could be just a short time away. It is not complicated and can be taught to just about anyone. Even children's classes can be very helpful for their understanding of how to bring calm focus to their minds and comfort to their souls.

Parents, children, teens, and all members of a family unit can benefit from Reiki. The family dynamic can be bound by entanglements that keep our energy from being free and clear. Our family energies are often extremely complex and convoluted to the point that we no longer know if this energy is even "mine." In relationships, we often stand in a hall of mirrors, not quite certain if what we see is a viable path or a reflection of someone else's projections. Reiki can help everyone in the family get clarity and return to their inner strength and light.

Today's stresses, which are arguably the most difficult in recent generations, affect even our youngest members of the family, who may be socially and energetically challenged because of pandemic protocols, social media, and screen projections, which are similar to the hall of mirrors analogy above, but even more distracting and deceptive to our younger generations. Reiki can help clear the biofield of energies that children and teens have picked up and this can often provide them with a renewed sense of self or a healthy tool to manage extreme stress.

Professional and elite athletes look to Reiki to help with habitual patterns in their mental, emotional, or physical game as they work to rebalance and shift how they use their energetic resources during practice, play, and competition.

My Reiki clients have included Olympic and elite gymnasts, runners, Olympic skaters and cyclists, PGA golf pros, football players, tennis pros, and dancers.

Military personnel, both active and retired, seek Reiki to assist with the extreme stress they experience. Reiki can be very helpful with PTSD and can recalibrate the energetic imprints when they are still feeling anxiety long after the crisis has ended. I see clients from all branches of the military. Reiki is recognized by the US Department of Veterans Affairs (VA) as a recommended complementary and integrative approach.

Caregivers—doctors, nurses, all types of medical personnel, first responders, home healthcare workers, and the like—seek Reiki to support their work and manage burnout symptoms. Compassion fatigue, which is often akin to post-traumatic stress disorder (PTSD), hits so many of our hardest-working caregivers to the point that some will feel the need to walk away from their jobs, from their heart's calling, as a form of self-preservation, because they are vulnerable to the traumatic work environment. Reiki can be revitalizing, as it lifts their biofield and releases them from the energetic imprints of other people's traumas, thus severing the cord to secondary traumatic experiences. This does not keep them from connecting with others, but it does give them a bit of distance to hold their space and vibrate higher in difficult times.

Patients who are dealing with the stresses of a diagnosed illness can benefit from the supportive energies of Reiki. Reiki promotes the relaxation response needed for the body to heal itself and energetic support for those undergoing treatments that can be challenging for the body, such as chemotherapy, radiation, or immunotherapies. Reiki can also help support those who are experiencing treatment fatigue or chronic fatigue syndrome, particularly when coming through a lengthy illness.

Reiki can be performed in hospitals, care/treatment centers, and before, after, and during surgery. Many hospitals, particularly teaching hospitals, have Reiki practitioners available at the patient's request, and some hospitals have programs available and will offer Reiki to patients as part of their recommended care. More will be discussed about this in later chapters.

Hospice and palliative care may offer Reiki for patients and families to bring calming peace during this sensitive period of serious illness and transition. Reiki can bring great comfort in the final stages of life for patients, families, and caregivers, and it is a lovely way to care for everyone involved. Reiki seeks to bring more love into the process of transitioning. If this therapy is not offered, patients and their families should be able to ask the hospice office; they will surely know how to connect the patient with a qualified and experienced Reiki practitioner who would be honored to work with them.

Reiki for animals can be a lovely healing experience for both the animal and their person. Most animals love Reiki and may even "ask" for its healing energies. If the animal is well enough and able to, have them move their physical body toward the practitioner's hands so the animal can "show" them where the healing energy is needed. Reiki, being intelligent energy, will know exactly what is needed and flow in the direction that is highest and best.

The plant kingdom loves Reiki, and it provides more energy to assist plants in growing and thriving. As climate challenges become more prevalent, Reiki healing can be very helpful in supporting the plants' innate power and life force within. We depend on the health of the plant kingdom for our own lives; how beautiful it is when we can call forth Reiki in service to the health and healing of Mother Earth.

Sensitive individuals will sometimes seek Reiki without a clear sense of why they feel called to this treatment. They feel an inner call to the work but are not fully aware of why. I want to speak a word of assurance for you: sometimes, the soul is calling for the healing that is needed, a supportive light that will move you further along your path. When the timing is right, lean in, and the path will alight for you.

Reiki—Care for the Soul

Reiki is often mistakenly considered to be a form of massage. This is incorrect. Massage will rub, knead, or manipulate the physical form to bring about the relaxation response. Reiki's touch does not do that. If the massage therapist is using Reiki, they will need to stop moving their hands to allow the flow of Reiki to do its work, without the force of physical movement. If the Reiki practitioner uses a gentle hands-on position, the position is held still as the energy flows into the one receiving it; there is no movement at all. And many will use no touch at all for the Reiki session, which is extremely powerful.

The confusion in calling Reiki a form of massage comes from the fact that it is regularly offered as supplemental training or continuing education units (CEU) for licensed massage therapists, like reflexology or acupressure.

However, in the case of reflexology or acupressure, we don't seem to confuse them with massage; they are clearly different modalities from massage. Reiki is more closely aligned with reflexology and acupressure than massage in how it is conducted.

So, if we cannot accurately call Reiki a form of massage, where does it fit into the current hierarchy of healing modalities? This is the challenge of vibrational healing or natural energy healing. A client once described Reiki after her session as "a massage from the inside, with light." This beautiful description works on many levels, for what is that "inside" part of the self that could be reached only with light? The soul.

Centuries of writings about the nature of the soul come to us through every religious belief system and philosophical school of thought. However, for our purposes, we will identify the soul as the eternal, immaterial part of the self that comes into embodiment to learn, grow, and return to its true home in spirit. The physical body is a dense form of matter, animated by the life of this immortal aspect of the self, the soul.

Reiki brings us back into alignment with the spark of the Divine that is present within all beings. Receiving Reiki helps to align us with our inherent life force, releasing built-up density, bringing us back to our authentic selves, and reconnecting us with our souls' guidance.

Reiki is sometimes referred to as a bridge of light. This light bridge clarifies the space—or seeming separation—that can appear to have been erected between us and our higher vibrational selves, our souls. The soul can never leave us, but the layers of density can give us the illusion of separation, bringing up feelings of incompleteness and a lack of wholeness. Many describe this as a disconnect, a lack of spiritual connection, or no longer feeling their inner guidance. Reiki clears out the heaviness of what was never ours to carry, releasing us from the weight of other people's energies, lower vibrations, and the effluvia of dysfunctional patterns that tend to build up in stressful times. Reiki is a bridge of light and a reconnection to the calling of the soul.

CHAPTER 2

Reiki Treatments and Sessions

There are several ways to receive Reiki from a certified practitioner. This may be referred to as a Reiki session or a Reiki treatment, which are used interchangeably. Reiki sessions are offered in the following modalities: in-person sessions, live virtual sessions, Reiki circles, and asynchronous/distance sessions. Each of these provides opportunities to receive Reiki in a manner that is convenient and comfortable for the recipient. We will examine each of these separately.

In-person Reiki Sessions

A private in-person Reiki session is usually scheduled with the Reiki practitioner in advance as an appointment at a particular office or center or an in-home session (yours or theirs). For those who are hospitalized or in long-term care facilities, Reiki practitioners (often Certified Medical Reiki Masters, CMRM) will meet the client for the appointment wherever required. In those cases, travel compensation may be appropriate.

Hopefully, the session will occur somewhere that is comfortable and puts the client at ease. Sometimes, that will not be found in the environment, such as in cases of hospitalization. Still, the practitioner should be able to help hold the energetic space in a healing vibration, wherever it is, caring for the soul of all concerned, even in challenging settings.

Intake Information

Intake information is the first bit of business for a private in-person session. Usually, paperwork is required so that both the client and the practitioner receive the information they need before the session begins. The intake form will also be used for live virtual sessions and possibly for asynchronous/distance sessions.

Each state has its own laws governing the use of what they commonly call "Alternative" Medicine. Some of the paperwork that needs to be filled out is to remain compliant with these laws. For example, in California, Reiki practitioners need to work within CA-SB577. So, a Reiki practitioner in California will gather basic client information, a statement of informed consent detailing what Reiki is, a privacy statement, and a form that provides practitioner information and details about their Reiki training and qualifications (see Appendix for an example of these forms).

What Would You Like from Your Session Today?

The Reiki practitioner is a neutral vessel through which the healing energy flows. My teacher, Raven Keyes, used to tell us that "we are the syringe, not the medicine." The syringe does not do the healing but delivers the medicine. In this way, the practitioner does not set the intention for the healing; the intention belongs to the one receiving the energy. The practitioner will ask the client about their intention for the session. Most understand the question and will be able to verbalize what they are working on, whether they are seeking healing in the physical body, mental health, emotional support, or spiritual comfort.

By talking about the issue at hand, you take responsibility for the energy that you have been holding and call forth the energetic links in their biofield/auric field to shift the dysfunctional patterns that created the issue. This is very effective in energy work.

Before the session, many clients may have a clear and specific intention for the healing. Others may find this difficult to discuss and would prefer to remain quiet. If the latter is the case, I encourage you to set a silent intention for your healing at the start of the session. It is never appropriate for the Reiki practitioner to set the intention for the recipient. That is a violation of the client's free will. The practitioner does not diagnose or prescribe and, therefore, does not set the goal for the client's healing.

The session belongs to the client; the Reiki is for you, and we are honored to bring that directly to YOU.

Touch or No Touch

Reiki, by definition, is a hands-on/light-touch energy healing modality. However, Reiki, being energy, is particularly suited to be administered in a no-touch manner by hovering slightly above the physical body. There should be a brief discussion about your comfort and your preference for receiving a touch or no-touch session.

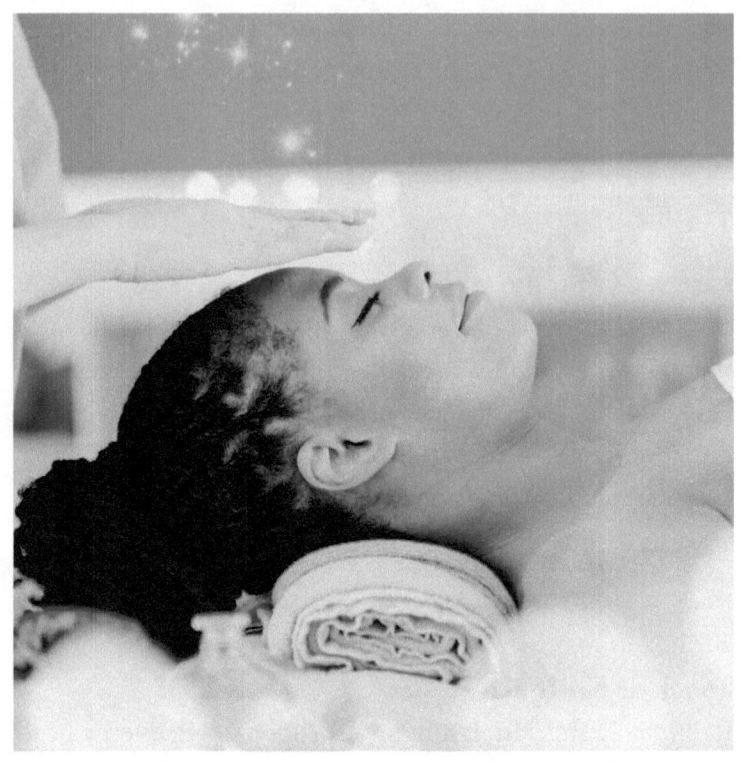

Receiving Reiki (Image: DragonImages & MLTorok/CanvaPro)

The preference is always up to you, and no practitioner will insist on placing hands on the physical body if 1. It is prohibited in the state or locality where the session is offered (some states mistakenly label Reiki as massage) or 2. It is not the recipient's preference. This is asked on my intake form, and I ask once again at the start of each session, "Just to be clear, are you comfortable if I place my hands on you during the session?"

You should feel free to express your preference and let your practitioner know if you change your mind during a session. Everyone should feel comfortable and at ease during their Reiki session. There is no diminished effect of the strength of Reiki, whichever is chosen: touch or no touch.

Comfort

The treatment room, whether at a professional center or in someone's home, should be energetically clear. You should feel comfortable and warmly welcomed. The space should put you at ease. Soft music will likely be playing, which helps to hold the vibrational space. A candle may also be lit, which helps to energetically cleanse the environment. Overall, the space should be peaceful and calming. Understandably, some sessions will take place in hospital rooms among bright lights, buzzing machinery, or any other uncontrollable environments. Do not worry; Reiki will bring the peace that is needed and meets you wherever you are.

There may be things you can do to make yourself feel more comfortable in an in-person Reiki session. Be sure to turn off your phone and any device that may disrupt your session. A digital shutdown is like a little vacation when you can take the time for yourself and unplug. Some are "on call" and will need to keep their phones on. If that is your case, discuss this with your practitioner so you can decide together how you will handle it if your device becomes a part of the session.

The recipient remains fully clothed during a Reiki session. Take your shoes off if that helps you relax. Take off anything that makes you feel uncomfortable—a tight ponytail, a watch, your glasses, or large jewelry, if they cause any discomfort. There is no requirement to remove anything unless it distracts you or makes you feel tension in any way. Reiki is not impaired by anything you are wearing, so do not worry about your watch, your shoes, or anything else. On or off, make yourself comfortable.

Reiki sessions can be given with the client lying down or in a seated position. Both have benefits. If lying down on a Reiki table is a challenge for you, ask the practitioner for a seated Reiki session. Many prefer this type of treatment, and it is not a problem at all.

The Reiki table is very similar to a massage table. However, there are some technical differences. A Reiki table has an opening at both ends so the practitioner can sit. This is not about the practitioner's comfort but about the level of their heart being in alignment with the client's flow of energy through the chakra column (energy centers). It is a clear heart/crown alignment.

Talking

Many clients ask about the level of conversation expected during a Reiki session. Sometimes, it is a great relief for the client seeking Reiki healing to have time without expectation for conversation, simply relaxing in a meditative state. But others will feel much better if they can talk about what is going on with them. In that case, some talk may feel appropriate during the session.

The practitioner, being fully engaged with the flow of Reiki throughout the session, will usually leave the level of talk to the client. Sometimes, I am inwardly guided to lead the client on a brief meditative journey to bring their conscious mind to a place somewhere out in nature where they can feel supported and free from the figuring mind.

If the client allows themself to relax fully, without the need to control or direct the energies, they will often experience multiple effects during a Reiki session.

That being said, I will often suggest that if there is anything the client is experiencing during their session that they feel they should share, please do, by all means.

Temperature Changes

During a Reiki session, temperatures can sometimes shift rather suddenly. Although my office thermostat will remain constant, the recipient or even the practitioner may feel energetic shifts as sudden changes in temperature. Be sure to share what you are experiencing during the session. Your practitioner may not be feeling the same changes as you.

I also offer my clients a top sheet or blanket to feel cozy on the table. Sometimes, that is enough to bring a bit more comfort to their personal space and allow them to relax just a little more. Be sure to ask for a blanket or to have the blanket removed if you find yourself getting too warm. Feel free to share whatever you are experiencing during the session.

Other Experiences

The following is a list of sensations or personal experiences clients have shared with me about what they felt during a Reiki session:

- peace and calm
- temperature changes
- a feeling of weightlessness or floating sensations
- a feeling of heaviness throughout the body/sinking into the table or chair
- seeing changing colors, patterns, or geometric shapes with their eyes closed
- tingling, pulsing, or vibrating sensations
- a sensation of bubbling effervescence
- shifts, jolts, or twitches

- memories that they had not thought about in decades
- pressure in various body parts
- scents (not from anything present in the physical surroundings) that brought up memories or familiar associations
- a sense that there were more people in the room, working with them (sometimes they have a sense of "who" they are)
- a sense of peace or an inner knowing about something that was troubling them or a concern they had
- a sense of being embraced by great love and light

Live Virtual Sessions

A live virtual session is one in which the practitioner and the client meet synchronously (at the same time) but in different places. This can be done using various video calling technologies, such as FaceTime, Zoom, Google Meet, Skype, etc.

The live virtual Reiki session is very similar to the in-person session. There is little to no "dilution" of the energy since the Reiki energy was not the practitioner's energy to begin with. Remember, the energy is channelled directly to the one receiving the healing, not filtered through the practitioner's energy system first. For this reason, any and all of the experiences listed above are possible for the one receiving a live virtual session, as well.

In a virtual setting, your practitioner will be holding space for the session, transmitting Reiki to you, wherever you happen to be, anywhere on the planet. Any resistance to this sort of healing is entirely in the minds of the people involved. Reiki healing energy is Divine energy and is unlimited in potential. If either the client or the practitioner has any misgivings about the quality of the energy given or received, it will undoubtedly be diminished. But this is true even during in-person sessions. Any limitation we place on the healing potential of Divine Presence Reiki is ours, not Reiki's.

Preparing Your Space for a Live Virtual Reiki Session
Before the appointment, you will want to consider where you will be for your session. This should be a space where you will be alone and uninterrupted (as much as possible). If you can, it is best to lie down, placing your screen (phone, laptop, tablet, etc.) at a distance or even across the room from you so the practitioner can see much of the body. You could be lying on a sofa, on the floor, or even on a bed. If you cannot lie down for whatever reason, a seated position is certainly acceptable as long as you can relax.

I have conducted virtual Reiki sessions with the recipient in their car on several occasions, even during workday lunch breaks. In that case, you will want to take a little time figuring out where to place the device so you are not holding it in your lap during the session. The device should be out of your hands and not resting on your body. Also, take a moment to consider the weather, as you don't want to be running the car's air conditioner for an hour or so. But sometimes, this happens, and we do the best we can. Reiki will not be stopped just because the car is idling. All is well.

Given the considerations of your space, you may want to light a candle to cleanse the space energetically. But this is not a requirement. There is no need for you to play music. Your practitioner will be able to do that for you from their end through your device's audio speaker.

If you are a parent of young children, you may want to enlist a sitter for your session so you can focus on your healing for the hour, or so. This will be a matter of scheduling your appointment for your benefit. Avoid scheduling your appointment during a toddler's nap, expecting them to sleep during their usual interval. The client will invariably be distracted, anxious, or called away from the session.

Although animals usually love participating in a virtual Reiki session, they tend to be somewhat disruptive. You should also discuss that possibility with your practitioner at the beginning, especially if it will be less obtrusive to have the animal freely move through the space. Personally, I find the animal will also receive the amount of Reiki that they need in the session and have no trouble with their movements. But it usually keeps the client just a little more consciously aware during their session.

During the Live Virtual Session
After the short discussion about your goals for the session, you will be encouraged to settle into relaxation. You may be guided in a meditation to help you relax. One of the benefits of the virtual Reiki session is that the client is usually already in a physical place of comfort; they are home, perhaps even in bed. This familiar environment may allow them to receive the Reiki energy more easily, as it flows without any resistance.

The experience of Reiki in a live virtual session is no different from an in-person session. You will have experiences similar to those you had in a face-to-face session. It can be quite a beautiful and healing experience. That is why spending a little time thinking about how best to prepare your environment is so important.

Reiki Circle/Reiki Share

Try out a sample Reiki session with an introduction to a Reiki Circle, sometimes called a Reiki Share. This is a community gathering of those who want to experience Reiki without committing to a private session. Although each Reiki Circle may have its own parameters, in general, it is where Reiki practitioners at all levels of experience, from Level I to Reiki Master, gather to give and receive Reiki. Each group member will receive Reiki, given by those who have been attuned. The person on the table may have three practitioners or up to thirty (I have experienced this once). The person receiving Reiki will have a shortened session, usually somewhere between ten and thirty minutes, with several practitioners at once.

These shortened sessions are usually no-touch/hands-off sessions, and they rarely lend themselves to individual consultations, as that is not the purpose. However, the energetic intensity from several practitioners at once is remarkable and certainly worth experiencing if you are looking for an introduction to Reiki.

When facilitating a Reiki Circle, I usually begin with a brief talk, a few minutes of introduction to Reiki, followed by a short, guided meditation to bring focus to the participants and to cleanse the energy field. We then proceed to the mini-Reiki sessions, often setting up multiple Reiki tables in the room, depending on the number in attendance. We agree on the length of time for each session, and then we begin.

At the end of the Reiki Circle, there is usually time to share your experiences and discuss Reiki in more detail. Reiki Circles can be a beautiful introduction to the work and a lovely way to connect with a community of like-minded individuals. Reiki Circles are also available online and may be found worldwide on social media platforms.

Asynchronous/Distance Healing Sessions

Reiki, being Divine and unlimited, is not bound by our limitations of time and space. Remembering that the practitioner is not the source of Reiki energy, it is easy to understand how we may receive a Reiki session asynchronously at a distance. These types of sessions do not require a common appointed time. The recipient does not need to be doing anything in particular while receiving this energy— you may be sleeping, or fully awake and going about your daily tasks, or anything in between.

There is usually some sort of communication before the session, where the recipient shares their intention for the healing with the practitioner, as discussed previously. The recipient is giving their full consent at this point. As a practitioner is never allowed to bypass the laws of free will, the person receiving the Reiki healing energy will always need to give their permission beforehand.

An asynchronous/distance session is extremely effective for those who cannot receive visitors, are traveling and unable to meet with their practitioner, or are too tightly scheduled to find a common time. Distance sessions can be a powerful way to receive Reiki during surgery if you cannot coordinate the presence of a Certified Medical Reiki Master in the operating room. Many clients report terrific results from these distance Reiki sessions, as the Reiki energy brings great support during challenging times.

Reiki in Hospitals and Care Centers (Medical Reiki)

In-person, live virtual, and asynchronous/distance sessions can be coordinated for those who are hospitalized or in care or treatment facilities of all types. Reiki can be of great assistance as it offers collaborative care and can support any and all forms of treatments or medications being given without contraindications. You can read more about Medical Reiki in Chapter 3, Integrative Medicine, Medical Reiki, and Clinical Settings.

***

Each Reiki session, no matter how it is delivered—in person, virtually, or asynchronously—will be a unique experience for the recipient. The Greek philosopher Heraclitus explained that because everything—the universe and rivers alike—is in motion, you cannot step into the same river twice. The river is always changing, and so are you.[2]

For this very reason, every time you step into the energetic river of Reiki, it will be a slightly different experience. Each session you receive clears your biofield and the accompanying heaviness, or density, a bit more, so the energy flows more freely. As the energy flows clearer, the healing work can go deeper. As the healing goes deeper, it clears your biofield a bit more, and so on.

It is also important to note that for that same reason, each practitioner will have a container for Reiki that flows a bit differently, as well. As with any healing relationship, you may find different results with different practitioners. More will be said about this in Chapter 5, Finding a Qualified Reiki Practitioner.

What Does the Recipient Do During a Reiki Session?

There is nothing for the recipient to actively *do* during a Reiki session. Some who are familiar with energy work will sometimes attempt to "help" the session by pushing with or pulling from the energy field. However, this rarely assists the practitioner and may, in fact, get in the way of what is highest and best. Just as the practitioner is a neutral delivery system (remember the syringe metaphor), the client should try to remain clear, to the degree that they are able. You have set your intention for the healing. Trust this, and let it go.

At the start of the session, open your heart and mind, then gently drop into the center of your being, here and now. Allow the energy to flow wherever it is needed, wherever it is highest and best. During a Reiki session, you are asked to simply relax and allow the flow of ki (chi, qi). In this way, a Reiki session, for the recipient, is very much like a meditation.

Your practitioner may sense that you need assistance in opening your heart and mind or getting out of the way of the energetic flow. They may invite you to bring your awareness to your breath, envision a beautiful place in nature, or see a great shining light flowing around you from above. These and many other meditative techniques may help you relax, step out of the way, and receive the flow of Reiki. Even if your practitioner does not invite you to do this, you can do this for yourself with great benefit.

If it is challenging to meditate or quiet the chatter of the figuring mind, know that Reiki can assist. Simply allow the energy to flow, repeating a gentle mantra with your inner voice while remaining inwardly focused. Any of the following, or creating something of your own, may assist:

- I am present, here and now—breathing in, breathing out.
- I am open to receiving healing light.
- I joyfully accept the healing energies.
- Reiki is love; love heals.
- Thank you.

Effects of a Reiki Treatment

Reiki reminds us of what peace, calm, and health feel like. As the ki (chi, qi) begins to flow more freely, it relaxes the physical, mental, and emotional bodies, making healing possible. Reiki is a personal experience, and the effects are wide and varied among recipients since everyone's needs are different. Overall, Reiki allows us to release stress and tension, allowing us to return to the strength of our own light—our true self.

Here is a short list of self-reported outcomes from my clients who have received Reiki:

Physical effects:
- relief from pain
- less physical tension and stress
- feeling lighter and more calm
- feeling more space within
- feeling refreshed
- better sleep
- increased energy levels
- improved recovery and speed of healing

- accelerated healing of fractures
- reduction in headaches and migraines
- reduction in arthritic pain
- relief of symptoms
- graduation from hospice

Mental and emotional effects:
- better moods
- reduced anxiety
- feelings of being supported
- feeling more optimistic, confident, and motivated
- reduction in mental chatter
- improved focus and mental clarity
- lifting of the "dark cloud"
- feelings of inner peace, balance, and harmony
- renewed sense of wellbeing

Spiritual effects:
- increased spiritual awareness
- feeling supported on the life path
- strengthened life force and personal empowerment
- feelings of wholeness and unconditional love
- deeper connection to inner wisdom and guidance
- support in the process of forgiveness and letting go
- increase in the presence of light
- alignment with the soul

As mentioned previously, on more than one occasion, clients have described the session as receiving a "massage for the soul" or a "massage from the inside."

Evidence-based research shows more specific outcomes, such as Heart Rate Variability, reduction in pain medications, and quicker recovery after surgery. Chapter 4,

Evidence-based Studies of Reiki's Effectiveness, discusses these studies in detail.

Although it would be irresponsible to describe Reiki as a miraculous healing modality, I cannot deny that miraculous healing has taken place with Reiki. Without false hope, denial, or naivety, the Reiki practitioner holds the space for the miraculous. Those seeking healing should remember that Reiki is unlimited in potential. Being the energy of Divine Universal light and love, Reiki *can* heal anything and everything.

Who Can Receive Reiki?

There are no restrictions on who can or cannot receive Reiki. As described earlier in this chapter, people of all ages and stages of life can benefit from this supportive healing energy. The same is true for the animal kingdom. Many also seek Reiki support for the beloved animals who share their homes.

Permission must be given for the session. An adult receiving Reiki must give their informed consent for the session. If the recipient is not yet an adult or one who is cared for by a legal guardian, it is the parent or guardian who will give permission for the Reiki session.

This is a good time to mention that young children, perhaps thirteen and under, may benefit from shorter sessions, like 30 minutes or so. Young children with smaller bodies may benefit from just a few minutes.

Are There Contraindications or Negative Side Effects from a Reiki Session?

There are no contraindications and no unhealthy side effects from a Reiki treatment. However, there may be positive outcomes to be aware of. For example, if you suffer from high blood pressure and take medication to control this issue, Reiki may, in fact, lower your blood pressure. In consultation with your prescribing doctor, your medication may need to reflect this healthy change. The same may be true for medications that deal with diabetes, fibromyalgia, depression, and so on. These are not negative side effects; they are the result of healing taking place. However, every Reiki recipient should know that Reiki used for specific diagnoses is best coordinated and used collaboratively. Let your doctor know that you are also taking Reiki treatments.

Unlike some treatment modalities, no "healing crisis" is associated with Reiki treatments or their aftermath. There is no release of toxins that need to be processed by the body or the liver. There should be no headaches or fatigue after a Reiki session. You may, however, feel extremely relaxed and may benefit from a short nap afterward, but this is not universally common. Most people feel energetically clear and quite ready to move on with their day.

If you feel unwell immediately after a Reiki session (within an hour or so), there may be a lingering energetic attachment. This is very uncommon, and it would be best to contact your Reiki professional to let them know what you are feeling. They can assist you at a distance to clear the last bit of energetic residue.

If this unusual feeling comes up more than an hour or so after your session, days or weeks after, then it is not from your Reiki session but something that is coming up from your thoughts or emotions that are not directly related to the Reiki clearing. Perhaps you are making changes in your life now that you feel the support of Reiki and the positive life force.

It is important to note how you feel after your Reiki session. You should immediately feel better and well—lighter, stronger, freer. Reiki healing is not something that develops later; it is immediate. After the session, if you remain in the flow, you may still receive further Reiki healing and guidance from your soul's growing light. Simply allow the ki (chi/qi) to flow.

Reiki can be a very effective resource on your healing journey and on your life path. As you shift and evolve throughout your life, there may be painful aspects to your growth and healing. Reiki does not cause growing pains but gives you the courage, space, and grace to shine a light into the shadows, healing the difficult places.

How Long Do the Effects of a Reiki Treatment Last?

Feeling light-filled and clear after your Reiki session is often a life-changing experience. It may remind you of what it feels like to be fully aligned with your soul. What a blessing! I liken it to getting another chance to hold the space of light in the world. And what a complex world it is. What you do *after* the session determines how long the positive effects of the Reiki session will stay with you. Remember, we are beings of free will who determine our outcomes. The law of free will governs all of humanity at all levels. It is our greatest strength and our greatest responsibility.

If you walk out of the session feeling terrific: light, clear, and strong, you will resonate with those frequencies, exponentially vibrating that out into the collective field. If, however, you get into your car and, just ten minutes later, are angered by another driver cutting in front of you, and fall back into old reactionary ways, you may call back into yourself something that vibrates at the level of rage. In this case, you are not bringing back exactly what was beautifully released by your Reiki session but something that energetically vibrates at the same lower frequency. The law of vibration is always at work: "Like vibrates like."

Of course, this is a fictitious example. I have not heard of this happening after a Reiki session in exactly this way. However, it reminds us that where our thoughts and our emotions go, energy flows. We are each responsible for the energies we release into the world. To that end, Reiki can be a terrific support in challenging times, particularly for those who are attempting to commit to a path of greater light and love. The healing path is met without resistance for those who work to align with healing energies in body, mind, and spirit. It is difficult to heal the body when the mind and spirit are toxic.

Reiki does not expect us to be perfect, hardly. But it does assist us in improving ourselves, raising our frequency, and learning to take responsibility for our personal atmosphere, our biofield. For clients who have aligned with these principles of energetic upliftment, the effects of a single Reiki session can last for weeks, months, or longer. Further, Reiki assists those who are working on a path of growth, helping them to have more patience and grace and to make healthier choices in all areas of their lives.

How Often Do I Need to Receive Reiki Treatments?

There are no requirements for a set number of Reiki sessions. As mentioned earlier, a single session can bring great upliftment. However, if you are on a path of healing and growth and feel that the session supports your journey, you may wish to return for additional sessions. Two or three sessions can be a terrific way to clear the heavy energies, raise your resonant frequency, and support a transformational path.

I have seen clients who are experiencing acute symptoms on a weekly or bi-weekly basis for a concentrated period. This may include those who are undergoing surgery, cancer treatment (chemotherapy or radiation), or are in the ICU. There are no limitations as to how often you can receive Reiki sessions. There are no wait periods required between Reiki sessions. Reiki cannot harm since it is Divine light and love. For example, I, like most serious Reiki professionals, give myself Reiki daily or even twice daily. More will be discussed about becoming "attuned" to Reiki so you can give yourself Reiki treatments in Chapter 5, Finding a Qualified Reiki Practitioner.

For those who are working on long-term health and growth, monthly Reiki sessions provide terrific support. Alternatively, I also have quite a few clients who come in seasonally, at the change of each earth-calendar season, for support. Of course, it is always up to you, and no Reiki practitioner would ever pressure you into sessions. I have some clients who return after a year or two to begin their next phase of growth or who are seeking Reiki support for a new challenge that has presented in their lives.

There are no long-term (or short-term) commitments with Reiki. Since Reiki is energy, I often tell my clients that they will "feel" when it is time to return for another session. I ask them to note how they feel after their session and encourage them to return when they no longer feel as clear, balanced, or light. Sometimes, it takes a little while to become sensitive enough to notice how your personal energy feels, but that will come in time with mindful practice.

CHAPTER 3

Care of the Soul in Clinical Settings

At some point in our lives, as human beings in human bodies, we will find ourselves in a doctor's care. Perhaps this will be quite often. It may be for us or for those we love. It may be for a small discomfort or a matter of life or death. Often, it is for something somewhere in between. For most of us, this brings up some level of concern or fear. Anxiety often accompanies our healthcare experiences; we even have a name for it: white-coat hypertension.

Larger health issues can be disorienting, moving us off-center as we grapple to regain our equilibrium amid "scary" diagnoses and even scarier treatment plans. We intellectually understand the importance of taking care of our mental and emotional health during challenging times such as these. Mental health professionals are often sought or services offered to those undergoing stressful life situations. Physicians understand the value of caring for the individual's physical, mental, and emotional health.

We have seen how a diagnosis does not necessarily mean the same result for everyone. Why would that be the case if the diagnosis had inevitable outcomes? And two people with the same treatment plans can also have different outcomes. Why would that be the case if the treatment always meant a cure? Obviously, there are other variables involved.

Variables affect results in all of life's situations. These variables could be the individual's mental state, emotional balance, or even the energy flowing through the biofield. Many will seek psychotherapy to assist them in handling the mental and emotional aspects during challenging times, and that is terrific. But how do we manage the energy of the etheric body and the surrounding biofield? Can we say we are taking care of our health if we are not tending to the biofield, spiritual energy, and caring for the soul?

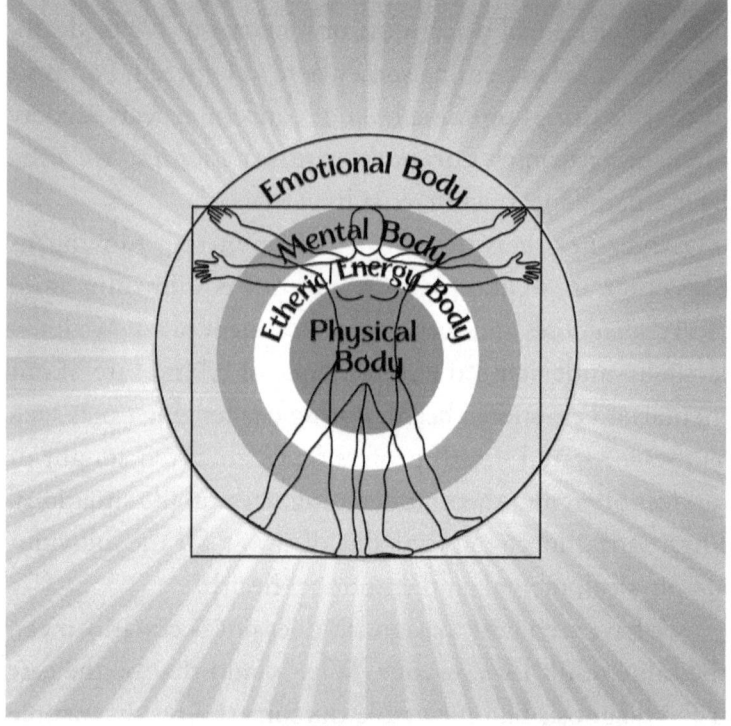

The Lower Bodies: The physical body + the biofield. The biofield surrounds the physical body in a 360-degree sphere, resonating throughout its environment. (MLTorok/CanvaPro)

Health encompasses the whole being. The disease may show symptoms at any one of those levels: body, mind, emotion, or spirit. Quite often, we seek care only for the relief of the symptoms, which is unlikely to bring true and full health. If our healthcare system does not care for the whole being, isn't it really a system of disease care?

Whole Health and Integrative Medicine

The American Board of Physician Specialties (ABPS) describes Integrative Medicine in the terms that were originally defined by Andrew Weil, MD, author and founder of the Andrew Weil Center for Integrative Medicine:

- A partnership between the patient and the practitioner.
- All factors that influence health, wellness, and disease are taken into consideration, including mind, spirit, and community, as well as body.
- Appropriate use of both conventional and complementary methods facilitates the body's innate healing response.
- Effective interventions that are natural and less invasive should be used whenever possible.
- Integrative medicine neither rejects conventional medicine nor accepts complementary therapies uncritically.
- Good medicine is based on good science. It is inquiry-driven and open to new paradigms.
- Alongside the concept of treatment, the broader concepts of health promotion and the prevention of illness are paramount.

- Practitioners of integrative medicine should exemplify its principles and commit themselves to self-exploration and self-development.

The Role of Spiritual Community

In the past, many people would find meaningful solace in their personal beliefs or support in their religious community. However, increasingly this is not the case in today's world.

According to research conducted by Gallup in 1973, 93 percent of the American population identified themselves as "religious," while five percent identified as not belonging to any particular belief system. Compared with recent times, in a 2024 study, 75 percent identified themselves as belonging to a religion, with 22 percent not belonging to any particular religion. Further studies also show that the religious community holds varying levels of importance for the individual within those with religious affiliations. In fact, in 2019, Gallup reported that less than 50 percent of Americans felt that religion was important to them. In 2023, church membership dropped well below that, at 45 percent. In summary, the majority of the American population who find themselves in hospital care will not have a spiritual support system available to them.

It is no longer appropriate to assume that the patient coming in for physical treatment is receiving mental/emotional support or spiritual care. Because Reiki is not dependent on any belief system or worldview, it is a particularly useful and effective way to care for the patient's spiritual or soul health without doctrine or dogma. The hospital or clinical treatment center is where Reiki shines.

The Role of Reiki in Integrative Healthcare

Reiki in medical and clinical settings provides the same effective healing outcomes that individuals experience in self-administered Reiki treatments and private sessions. More than 800 hospitals in the United States offer Reiki as a complementary part of their treatment protocols, and more than sixty US hospitals have adopted Reiki as part of patient services.[3]

Reiki professionals, nurses, and therapists with professional training are available in many medical and clinical settings to offer Reiki as an integrated part of a patient's healthcare journey. In fact, many nurses are offered Reiki training as part of their continuing education units (CEU). With some knowledge and understanding, you can request this supportive, collaborative care for yourself and those you love whenever needed.

In a 2024 presentation before the Certified Medical Reiki Masters and Medical Reiki Works Board of Directors, Sheldon Marc Feldman, MD, Director of Breast Surgery at Montefiore Einstein Cancer Center and Alyson Moadel-Robblee, PhD, Director of BOLD Program – Psychological & Integrative Oncology presented an update about their current Reiki clinical trial. At the time of this writing, they are investigating the effectiveness of Medical Reiki for women undergoing breast cancer treatments and the impact on quality of life, medical recovery metrics, and cortisol levels. This groundbreaking research is in cooperation with Medical Reiki Works.

During his presentation, Dr. Sheldon Marc Feldman discussed his wholehearted first-hand experiences with the power of Reiki to bring exceptional outcomes to his patients for many years, particularly with his work with Raven Keyes, founder of Raven Keyes Medical Reiki International. Dr. Feldman presented six ways that Reiki assists the patient in his care:

- during medical preparation—labs, x-rays, medical evaluations
- education, anticipation, expectations
- psychological/emotional/spiritual anxiety
- acceptance of loss: breast, femininity, sexuality, identity as nurturer
- teaching—serious illness as an opportunity for change
- helping to create space for health and wellness to become a priority[4]

It is very important to re-state here that Reiki is NOT a cure or a treatment *for* any specific ailment, disease, or diagnosis. However, adding Reiki as an integrative part of your care can beneficially assist your whole person on a healing journey and those who care for you in body, mind, and spirit. Since there are no harmful effects of a Reiki treatment, and many report deep relaxation and beneficial results from sessions, it is advised that you talk with your doctor about including Reiki in your treatment plan. This is particularly helpful when the diagnoses and the prescribed treatments bring a certain amount of stress and anxiety.

Health Insurance

The National Institutes of Health (NIH.gov) houses Reiki within its umbrella, the National Center for Complementary and Integrative Health (NCCIH). This is the lead federal agency for scientific research on the usefulness and safety of complementary and integrative medicine techniques. They describe Reiki as being safe, with no known negative side effects. They acknowledge the current lack of high-quality scientific studies that have proven the effectiveness of biofield therapies, Reiki being one of them. However, many smaller studies have been conducted worldwide, and several current double-blind, randomized studies are presently in trials. We will review some of the Reiki research in Chapter 4, Evidence-based Studies of Reiki's Effectiveness.

At the time of this writing, health insurance companies will cover Reiki treatments in a way that is similar to other therapies, like physical therapy, chiropractic, massage, or acupuncture. If your primary physician provides a referral for the treatment, it may be covered. You should check if your plan covers what is often called Complementary/Alternative Medicine (CAM) therapies or Complementary/Integrative Healthcare (CIH). Currently, insurance coverage for Reiki sessions is usually a reimbursement, so your practitioner will need to provide a proper and detailed receipt for your payment, which could then be submitted to your insurance company for reimbursement. Find out what needs to be included on the receipt to avoid any paperwork hiccups later.

Also, Reiki may be covered if your insurance provides you with a Healthcare Savings Plan (HSP), which allows you to use your "banked" funds for personalized wellness treatments without a referral.

Suppose your health insurance program covers complementary/alternative medicine (CAM) or Complementary/Integrative Healthcare (CIH) modalities. In that case, there may be certain restrictions on the provider's qualifications:

the level of professional training, licensing, or even the clinical setting where the treatment occurs. Research these stipulations before seeking a session if insurance coverage of this work is important to you.

If you are seeking Reiki treatment in a hospital setting, it may be covered by your insurance if it is a hospital-affiliated program. A team of hospital volunteers may also offer Reiki. There may be out-of-pocket fees associated with this sort of hospital call, or it may be offered free by volunteers. Fees will vary depending on your circumstances and locale. Simply ask for the details. Asking one of the nurses or a local Reiki practitioner in your area is a good place to start for in-hospital sessions.

The Veterans Association

The Veteran's Association (VA.gov) published *Passport to Whole Health* (2022/2024), which dedicates Chapter 17, "Energy Medicine: Biofield Therapies," to an in-depth analysis of biofield therapies, including Reiki.[5]

In this very thorough document, the VA describes how the time has come to commit to treating the whole person rather than just the disease. They offer the following diagram to visualize the need for a holistic approach to healthcare, and really, it is a formula for healthcare meeting wellness:

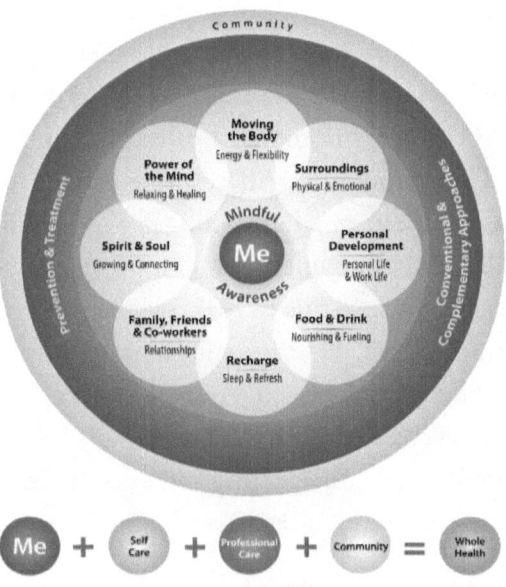

Conventional and complementary approaches to healing (Used under fair use: https://www.va.gov/WHOLEHEALTH/circle-of-health/index.asp)

The Veteran Association's "Whole Health" program includes every aspect of a person—"body, mind, spirit, and relationships with others. Physical well-being is important, but it is just the tip of the iceberg."[6]

These aspects of the self are very similar to the principles of Integrative Medicine that were presented earlier in Chapter 2, Reiki Treatments and Sessions.

The Veteran's Association's "Whole Health" website describes studies that show the number of veterans who look to Complementary/Integrative Health (CIH) approaches in their healthcare. A deeper look into a study in Hawaii of 401 veterans with chronic pain, non-cancer-related, found that 82 percent were using CIH modalities.[7]

According to a 2012 National Health Interview Survey, 73 percent of those interviewed have seen a practitioner for energy healing in their lifetime, while 43.5 percent had seen a practitioner for energy healing in the past twelve months. These studies have determined that even though one-third of American adults will seek CIH modalities for their healthcare as supplemental support, 40 percent of those will not disclose this to their primary care doctor.[8] It was determined that these patients kept the information to themselves because the doctor did not initiate the conversation and never asked. And the patient was fearful that the doctor would make disparaging remarks or ridicule them for seeking something "alternative."

Patient-driven Healthcare

It is time to put the term "alternative" away; it does a great disservice to its meaning. Alternative usually means that there is a choice between two. This or that. Regarding alternative medicine, it means the "other," untested, whacky, or woo-woo option. Patients do not necessarily want to defend their choices to the scientist in the lab coat who has never tried Reiki. This is why it is so important for Reiki practitioners who want to assist in bringing Reiki into hospitals to first offer it to doctors, nurses, and hospital personnel so they become familiar with what Reiki is…and what it is not. Reiki is better identified as integrative or collaborative care, and many programs are slowly switching their designations, so be on the lookout for both terms.

As individuals begin to assert their freedom over their healthcare choices, the institutions created to care for them will respond in kind. Western medicine, which is used to looking solely into microscopes and numbers on charts, will increasingly look into our eyes and see the windows to the soul—finding the care that is needed beyond the cellular level and treating the whole person at the energetic level. Do not get weary; just keep talking about your health goals and keep asking for what you need on your healing journey.

Reiki in Hospitals

Hospitals can locate a qualified Reiki practitioner, even if they don't yet have an integrated Reiki program. Quite often, trained practitioners are available through the spiritual care wing of the hospital or Reiki-trained chaplains. This is a terrific opportunity to experience Reiki as long as they are properly and fully trained. For more on this, see Chapter 5, Finding a Qualified Reiki Practitioner.

A Reiki program, often housed within an Integrative Care wing of the hospital, will usually have free or low-cost Reiki practitioners who can be scheduled to give Reiki treatments. If these practitioners are scheduled to see many patients in a short amount of time, the sessions may be shortened to just a few minutes, anywhere between ten and thirty minutes or so. However, a hospital with a full-service Reiki program may be able to offer a bit more. Teaching hospitals regularly have programs in integrative medicine, which offer Reiki, among other biofield healing modalities.

One of the most Reiki-forward hospitals in the country at the time of writing this book is Hartford Hospital in Connecticut. Their benchmark program, the Integrative Medicine Program, was officially launched in 1999 through a series of Women's Health Services, Cardiology, Orthopedics, and Oncology projects by offering wellness programs like Reiki to patients, families, and staff. Careful data collection measured overwhelming positive outcomes in pain reduction, anxiety relief, and patient satisfaction. From December 1999 to December 2000, they conducted a yearlong study which indicated that Reiki improved patient outcomes in the following ways:

- sleep improvement by 86 percent
- pain reduction by 78 percent
- nausea reduction by 80 percent
- anxiety reduction during pregnancy by 97 percent

For the past twenty-four-plus years, Hartford Hospital has been offering Reiki to every patient from the beginning, at admissions, through pre- and post-op, during surgery, and at any time at the request of the patient, family members, or caregivers. They also offer Reiki to inpatients, outpatients, and their families. Hartford Hospital reports that, overall, Reiki patients need less anesthesia, experience less bleeding during surgery, require fewer pain medications, and have shorter hospital stays.

The following is a short list of hospitals currently using Reiki as a part of an integrated approach to healthcare for patients, families, and their caregivers, along with the year they began implementing the program, where applicable:

In the United States:
- New York Presbyterian Hospital - Columbia University Medical Center Campus, NY (1995)
- Columbia University Medical Center, Integrative Therapies Program for Children with Cancer, NY (1997)
- Sharp Memorial, San Diego, CA (1998)

- Memorial Sloan Kettering Cancer Center, NY (1999)
- Children's Hospital, Boston, MA (1999)
- Dana Farber Cancer Institute, MA (2000)
- Yale New Haven Children's, CT (2006)
- Yale New Haven, CT (2008)
- Duke Integrative Medicine, Durham, NC (2007)
- Brigham and Women's Hospital, Boston, MA (2009)
- Montefiore Einstein Cancer Center, NY
- California Pacific Medical Center, San Francisco, CA
- George Washington University, Medical Center, Washington, DC
- York Hospital, York, ME
- Washington Hospital Center, Washington, DC
- Saint Joseph Hospital, Nashua, NH
- Harvard University, Boston/Cambridge, MA
- MD Anderson Cancer Center – University of Texas, Houston
- Cedars Sinai, Los Angeles, CA
- Mayo Clinic Health System, multiple locations worldwide

Cedars Sinai teaches Reiki classes every Wednesday for staff, patients, families, and the community. On their website, they acknowledge that caregivers are giving all day long. The hospital wants to take care of them with Reiki.

Mayo Clinic teaches Reiki in its hospital chapels on multiple campuses. It offers this service to staff, families, and the community who want to learn. The clinic is also conducting evidence-based clinical trials on the use of Reiki for hematology/oncology cancer patients, which began in the second half of 2023.

In Canada:
- University Health Network – Princess Margaret Hospital, Toronto, Ontario
- Université De Moncton, Moncton, Nouveau-Brunswick

In the United Kingdom:
- University College London hospitals, NHS, London
- Kings Mill Hospital – Nottinghamshire
- Southampton University Hospitals NHS, Southampton
- Aintree University Hospitals NHS, Liverpool
- Wallace Cancer Care, Cambridge
- South Tees Hospitals NHS, Middlesbrough
- Newham University Hospital NHS, London
- Great Ormond Street Hospital, London

Interestingly, many members of the UK Reiki Federation are licensed/practicing doctors and Reiki Masters.

It is also worth noting that these lists are incomplete and subject to change, but I hope they demonstrate how Reiki is recognized worldwide and how many medical facilities offer Reiki in the US, Canada, and the UK, as well as hospitals in Australia, Germany, Switzerland, New Zealand, Mexico, Chile, Argentina, Brazil, Spain, and Portugal. For a list of Reiki resources, go to www.reikiintegrativemedicine.com.

Reiki and Surgery

Pre- and post-op Reiki is a terrific way to receive the relaxation response that promotes healing surrounding one's surgery. These sessions can also be given at a distance. Still, with a little planning, you can have the energetic support of a Reiki professional accompany you to the hospital—meeting you at your check-in, sitting with you throughout the preparations or pre-op, and being there afterward, to clear your energy field of any mis-qualified energies that have been picked up in the biofield while you were unconscious. All of this is beautiful healing support.

Reiki professionals can also receive advanced training in "Medical Reiki," which gives them additional instruction and practice in giving Reiki in the operating room *during* surgery. Raven Keyes, author of *Medical Reiki*, taught her students that Reiki activates the parasympathetic nervous system, inducing calm, creating balance, and priming the body to better receive medical treatments prescribed by doctors and administered by nurses, which are necessary to combat disease. Receiving Reiki during surgery gives the patient an added ray of light throughout the surgery that allows the practitioner to hold space for the soul during the procedure.

Raven Keyes Medical Reiki International (RKMRI) trains and certifies Reiki Masters to the professional gold standard for bringing Reiki to the operating room. In development with Dr. Sheldon Marc Feldman, Raven Keyes created professional protocols for bringing Reiki professionals safely and unobtrusively into surgery. The Reiki practitioner sits on a stool, usually at the patient's head (next to the anesthesiologist or somewhere nearby but out of the way). They are silent and inwardly focused the entire time. The Medical Reiki practitioner stays the entire length of the surgery. If needed, they may step out briefly to use the restroom, but they return to their stool, silent and inwardly focused. Nurses or attending physicians may leave the surgery or be relieved by others, but your Reiki practitioner will remain with you, sending Divine light throughout.

Protocols for a Reiki practitioner to attend surgery vary from hospital to hospital and surgeon to surgeon. At the time of the writing, it is unlikely to be offered Reiki in surgery directly by your doctor or hospital unless you are fortunate enough to be in one of those listed above. However, everyone has a right to the care they seek.

So where do you start? It begins with the patient's request. Let your surgeon know that you want to have a Reiki practitioner in the surgery with you. And start from there. You can also find more information at www.ravenkeyesmedical-reiki.com and www.ReikiIntegrativeMedicine.com.

Reiki in Clinical Settings

Reiki accompanies medical treatments of all sorts, including outpatient surgeries, procedures, chemotherapy, radiation, dialysis, long-term care centers, palliative care, hospice, and all others. Reiki is non-invasive, fully portable, needs no tools or equipment, and can be brought into any office or clinical setting. In the same way, you might request a practitioner to visit you in the hospital; you can seek assistance at or during any upcoming treatment. Given my training, I am partial to those who have been well-trained in medical or clinical Reiki by professional schools, such as Raven Keyes Medical Reiki. More will be discussed about how to find a Reiki Professional in Chapter 5, Finding a Qualified Reiki Practitioner.

Reiki can also assist in the long haul of recuperation, particularly where the patient is experiencing treatment fatigue, as Reiki can rejuvenate and uplift energies. Reiki is deeply relaxing and creates a sense of well-being. This is a relaxation that goes beyond rest, sleep, or other bodywork techniques, for Reiki taps into life force energy to balance and energize the parasympathetic nervous system to promote the healing response. In fact, Reiki can assist those who suffer from insomnia or find it difficult to shut off the racing mind and anxious thoughts that keep them awake. In this way, Reiki can be a terrific complementary healing technique, in collaboration with other healing treatments one may be prescribed by their doctor or in ongoing care.

Reiki in Palliative Care and Hospice

Since Reiki is a gentle, non-invasive form of care, it is well-suited in situations where the individual has been diagnosed with a chronic or life-threatening illness or is seeking end-of-life care because while it is not a curative treatment, mental, emotional, and spiritual healing usually accompanies Reiki treatment. Informal studies show that Reiki in ongoing palliative care can help with the anxiety that often accompanies long-term and life-changing diagnoses and bring calm to the patient, their loved ones, and their caregivers. Reiki, being the presence of love, can help those who are at any stage of anticipatory grief or bereavement: denial, anger, bargaining, depression, or acceptance. Reiki can envelop the individual in a sense of immediate care that profoundly benefits them on all levels—mental, emotional, and spiritual. This can also help to ease physical discomforts.

Each of us experiences many losses in our lifetime, and many will find themselves walking with grief and its accompanying symptoms: sleep disruptions, changes in appetite, digestive discomfort, muscle tension, nausea, fatigue, hyper-vigilance, feelings of regret, and so on. During terminal illness and end-of-life experiences, we can find ourselves moving through the grieving process on at least three different levels:

- Regret for where we are now
- The loss of what life was like in the past
- The loss of a future that will not be

Connecting to the strength of our inner light, Reiki can bring us back to the center of our being, in the here and now, feeling the presence of love and its higher vibrations. After a Reiki session, many feel the expansion of their inner space, where they have more capacity to handle the experiences surrounding them. I have been honored to hold space for people with Reiki and have seen the calm strength that can grow from within during such challenging times.

Palliative care and hospice programs often have Reiki practitioners who are available to assist at any stage, from diagnosis through bereavement, and are helpful for anyone needing support. These types of sessions can be facilitated in hospitals, hospice homes, skilled nursing facilities, and private homes. Simply ask for assistance in locating an appropriate Reiki practitioner.

Reiki for Caregivers

Taking care of someone else is often an exhausting job. I mean that literally. In the way that most people care for others, they pour their energetic resources (their time and life force) into the person needing assistance. No matter how much you love them, if you are giving from this finite place, you will exhaust your inner resources. You will be exhausted. Visualize pouring a glass of water into another glass. One will always be less than full if you are giving the water from a limited source.

We are often taught that this is what it means to love someone; we give ourselves away in service to others. You give to your family, then you go to work and give to the patients who need you, you give to the neighbor who needs some help, you give to the charities that so desperately need, you give and give. No one seems to have enough, so you keep giving. Then you come home, and you hope that someone is there to give to you, to fill you back up. What if they, too, are empty? Or perhaps there is no one there at home? Your glass may be empty.

If this were a bank account, numerically keeping track of your energetic resources, you would be overdrawn or in debt. In this limited scenario of finite resources, there just isn't enough. This is where stress and anxiety can take their toll, sometimes leading us to make unhealthy choices that may provide a modicum of short-term relief: forms of escape, checking out, isolation, unhealthy foods, drugs, alcohol, and so on. How long can a good-hearted caregiver go on in this way? Trying to balance our energies with finite resources, we become overwhelmed by debt-consciousness, always seeking where we can get more of what we think we are lacking. Exhausting, isn't it?

Reiki may be the answer for caregivers to become care receivers. Reiki is not a transfer of energy—one person moving energy to another or transferring energetic funds to different places of the body. No. Reiki is given and received from a place of abundance, a place of limitless supply—infinitely connected and unconditionally available. It comes from an unlimited source.

The Reiki practitioner does not send out their own energy, as that would create an imbalance for the practitioner. Reiki is given from a place of fullness. And that is unlimited in potential. Caregivers who learn to use Reiki for themselves may find the inner resources to continue with their challenging work while maintaining full energy stores. Whether you are a professional or personal caregiver, or both, Reiki may assist you in keeping the glass full, no matter how much you give to others. There has been much research done on Reiki and burnout syndrome. This will be addressed in the next chapter.

CHAPTER 4

Evidence-based Studies of Reiki's Effectiveness

At the first-ever World Health Organization (WHO) Traditional Medicine Global Summit in August of 2023, the European Regional Director gave a stirring speech summarizing the work that was accomplished during this groundbreaking convention:

> *Together, we have gently shaken up the status quo that has, for far too long, separated different approaches to medicine and health. By taking aim at silos, we are saying we will collaborate all the more to find optimal ways to bring traditional, complementary, and integrative medicine well under the umbrella of primary health care and universal health coverage... We have reiterated how crucial it is to get better evidence on the effectiveness, safety and quality of traditional and complementary medicine. That means innovative methodologies for assessing and evaluating outcomes.*[9]

Reiki research is in its adolescent stages, as there has not been much interest in funding a technique that anyone can learn, do themselves, and costs very little. Investment in large-scale research usually means that there are potential monetary gains somewhere down the road. That will probably not be the case for something as natural and free as Reiki.

Nonetheless, quality studies have been completed and continue to be conducted. As of this writing, there are 140 Reiki studies and research papers listed on the Center for Reiki Research website (www.centerforreikiresearch.com), going back to 1989. And those who say that there is no evidence for Reiki's effectiveness are ill-informed and, perhaps, reveal a bias against integrative medicine. The National Center for Complementary and Integrative Health/National Institutes of Health (NCCIH.NIH.gov) and The Center for Reiki Research (centerforreikirsearch.org) maintain databases for Reiki research, which is becoming an important topic as Western medicine begins to take a long look at wellness. The studies and peer-reviewed articles are growing in numbers each year, and the evidence is mounting—Reiki works.

Below is a summary of just some of the most impressive evidence-based studies that have been conducted worldwide to date:

Results of a Single Reiki Session

In 2019, the *Journal of Alternative and Complementary Medicine* published the findings of "A large-scale effectiveness trial of Reiki for physical and psychological health."[10]

The objective of this study was to evaluate multiple levels of physical and psychological health, as self-reported before and after a single Reiki session, in private practice settings. This single-arm study also evaluated the data collection process of qualitative feedback for future studies.

The study utilized ninety-nine trained and certified Reiki Masters from all over the United States who provided common information to their clients about the study. The clients self-reported qualitative measures before and after their Reiki session (45–90 minutes). A total of 1411 sessions were conducted, and qualitative measurements were evaluated and included in the final analysis. This study validated statistically significant improvements for every measurement, including positive effects/mood, negative effects/mood (pain, drowsiness, tiredness, nausea, appetite, shortness of breath, anxiety, and depression), and overall well-being. The measurements proved to be positive and statistically significant on all criteria.

Recovery for Burnout Among Professionals

In 2011, a study was published in *Biological Research for Nursing*, which measured the "Immediate effects of Reiki on Heart Rate Variability, cortisol levels, and body temperature in health care professionals with burnout." This small-scale study of twenty-one healthcare professionals showed that Reiki, over placebo (what is commonly called "sham" Reiki in blind studies), produced a significant increase in Heart Rate Variability (HRV), and "these results suggest that Reiki affects the parasympathetic nervous system when applied to health care professionals with" burnout syndrome.[11]

More recently, also on the subject of burnout, the *International Journal of Advanced Multidisciplinary Research and Studies* published findings from a 2019–2020 study, "The effects of Reiki treatment on mental health professionals who are at risk of burnout." This was a much larger study, with 450 initial participants and 346 completing the training. The participants were given training in using Reiki. They received ten to fourteen days of training with a Reiki Master in accordance with the standards of practice from the International Center for Reiki Training (ICRT). Of the participants, 82 percent reported increased energy levels, and 59 percent reported regular use of Reiki therapy at home. All caregivers reported a sense of becoming more active participants at their workplace after receiving Reiki training. The conclusion of this study reports that Reiki shows a lessening of burnout symptoms "among experts dealing with patients on the spectrum."[12]

Support for Caregivers

In a 2012 study that was funded by the Seattle Children's Hospital Institutional Intramural Funds for Excellence, researchers also decided to train people who had previously been unfamiliar with Reiki. This pilot program created a hospital-based Reiki training program for caregivers of hospitalized pediatric patients. This was a small study of seventeen families, and the goals were realized in that the families were given the tools to use Reiki to benefit their child by improving comfort (76 percent did), providing relaxation (88 percent did), and pain relief (41 percent did). All family participants reported the added benefit of participating actively in the child's care. This study became the foundation of the pilot program for an ongoing hospital-based Reiki training program for caregivers.[13]

Going a little further into the healing effects of Reiki for individuals caring for cancer patients, *Complementary Therapies in Medicine* published a study conducted in May

2021 called "Effect of Reiki on the stress level of caregivers of patients with cancer: Qualitative and single-blind randomized controlled trial." Primary caregivers of cancer patients were randomly divided into two groups: those who would receive Reiki and those who would receive "sham" Reiki sessions. Those in the Reiki group were in sessions, receiving Reiki at seven main chakras/energy centers and two additional positions at a frequency of once a week for six weeks. The caregiver strain index (CSI) score dropped significantly for the Reiki group—from 10.09 before Reiki to 6.90 after Reiki. The placebo/"sham" Reiki group's CSI score went up from 9.40 before "sham" Reiki to 9.80 after "sham" Reiki. Of course, without any negative side effects reported, the qualitative statements of the Reiki participants were quite remarkable. Here are a couple of statements that are noted in the study:

• "I am not the same person before and after the session. I am sleeping now; what could be better than this?"
• "I felt a positive flow of energy in my body, in my thoughts, and in my mind. Reiki made me think positively and calmly."
• If you remember, I said that my neck was stuck because I did not sleep while I was waiting at the bedside of my patient at night. Now, there is none. I have abnormal blood pressure. Basically, my systolic blood pressure would not be lower than 140mmHg. I am surprised that it dropped and remained low with each session."

- Talking about giving Reiki to her partner who is hospitalized: "That warmth will spread to his body as we have, his muscles will relax, and he will learn to stop thinking, so he will experience such an unspeakable, spiritual maturity. This is also the case for any disease. I think it should be tried. I think Reiki should be part of the treatment." [14]

Use in Patient Care

A study published in *EXPLORE: The Journal of Science and Healing*, conducted between February and March of 2022, involved three groups of 52 stage III and IV cancer patients receiving palliative care, for a total of 156 participants. In "The effect of acupressure or Reiki interventions on the levels of pain and fatigue of cancer patients receiving palliative care: A randomized controlled study," patients were given either Reiki, acupressure (a form of hands-on energy healing based on the flow of chi and Chinese meridians), or nothing but standard care for the control group.

Reiki or acupressure was given to the intervention groups for eight sessions of twenty minutes each—twice a week for four weeks. The study was designed to collect data on a patient description form, an analgesic follow-up form, the Numeric Pain Rating Scale, and the Brief Fatigue Inventory. The results of this study showed that compared with the control group, a significant reduction was seen over time in the levels of pain, analgesic use, and fatigue in the groups receiving either Reiki or acupressure treatments. [15]

A 2023 study in *EXPLORE: The Journal of Science and Healing* evaluated Reiki for patients undergoing surgery. In "The effect of Reiki on anxiety, fear, pain, and oxygen saturation in abdominal surgery patients: A randomized controlled trial," researchers studied ninety-three participants who were divided into three different groups: Reiki, "sham" Reiki, and a control group. Ultimately, this study showed that surgical fear, anxiety levels, and pain decreased with the Reiki group. As well, levels of oxygen saturation increased overall with the Reiki group patients.[16]

After the study, the researchers ultimately recommended that since Reiki is inexpensive, safe, effective, and easy to apply, nurses should give patients Reiki as a part of their care when patients are undergoing abdominal surgery.

The March 2025 issue of the *Journal of Pain and Symptom Management* published an "Evaluation of a Reiki Volunteer Program within Two Cancer Infusion Centers." This two-year study ran between March 2022 and February 2024. A diverse group of participants received short (15 – 20 minute) Reiki sessions during outpatient cancer infusion treatments (e.g., chemotherapy). 392 Reiki sessions were provided to 268 unique patients. Data was collected before and after the treatments, using the Edmonton Symptom Assessment System measuring symptom levels such as pain, fatigue, anxiety, nausea, and overall well-being. There were significant (95% CI, confidence intervals) improvements in all symptoms. There was also a high level of satisfaction with this positive healing experience.[17] It is interesting to note that these sessions were merely mini-sessions, lasting just 15 – 20 minutes in length. These sessions were usually short, with impressive outcomes.

The Future of Reiki Research

Research results continue to consistently show that Reiki is effective in cooperative care for those undergoing procedures and treatments. High-quality double-blind trials are being conducted at major hospitals in the United States, including New York Presbyterian. The results of which we eagerly await. Until that time when we have conclusive evidence, Reiki remains at the level of patient-initiated care—in this case, meaning that the patient may need to request Reiki as part of their care, until it is a standard offering of every hospital desiring to offer patient-centered healing practices along with disease management.

The Center for Reiki Research (CRR) is a non-profit organization dedicated to Reiki research and education. They are an excellent resource for current studies about Reiki. Find more at www.centerforreikiresearch.com

CHAPTER 5
Finding a Qualified Reiki Practitioner

Many different forms of Reiki are practiced in the world today, perhaps close to a hundred different types in all, according to some sources. The most prevalent form of Reiki, and the one we are primarily focusing on in this book, is the practice that comes from the Usui lineage and is often referred to as Usui Reiki or Usui Reiki Ryoho. The Japanese word "ryoho" is translated as method or system. If you are interested in experiencing Reiki—receiving a session or finding a practitioner near you—it may be helpful to learn a bit about Reiki training and your options.

Understanding Reiki Training

Reiki training is a comprehensive process. The experiential classes are taken at three degrees or levels: Reiki I, Reiki II, and Reiki III. Although a student or practitioner may certainly share Reiki with others before the training is complete, professional training is not fully complete until the three levels of Reiki are attained.

Although you are learning *about* Reiki by reading this book, you are not receiving Reiki training by reading this book. Reiki cannot be learned from books alone, by taking asynchronous (self-study) online workshops, or solely by watching videos. Although these may be lovely supplemental materials as *part* of your training, they are not considered the professional standards for Reiki training. Some international professional organizations will not recognize individuals as qualified Reiki Masters if their training is fully asynchronous without the *presence* of a certified Reiki Master Teacher.

Reiki is high-vibrational energy, many will say Divine energy, and is passed in the presence of the Reiki Master Teacher to the Reiki student in a process called "attunement." This beautiful word resonates with the musical idea of tuning an instrument or orchestra to play together, fully connected and resonating as one.

Attunements (also called empowerments, activations, placements, or ignitions—in certain traditions) are the process by which Reiki energy is initiated, clarified, and amplified. Attunements are initiated by well-qualified Reiki Master Teachers who have substantial energetic clarity and experience.

The attunement process is a sacred mystical experience, as the energy is received directly from the octave of the spiritual plane. The teacher, at the level of the physical plane, is holding space and creating the container for the spiritual activation of the energetic system, which happens at a much higher vibrational level. In other words, the teacher is doing their part of the attunement ritual at the physical level, but the activation of the energy is completed from the highest spiritual level—the Divine presence.

This is also why attunements given asynchronously, without the teacher's presence, are not ideal and, perhaps, energetically muddy. The presence of the Master Teacher provides a level of strength and protection for the students during the attunement. Professional Reiki organizations recommend that one who seeks a qualified practitioner should be sure that their attunements were conducted in the actual "presence" of the teacher—whether in person or online.

According to traditional standards, four attunements are given at Reiki I, two attunements are given at Reiki II, and the final/Master attunement is given at level III training.[18] These attunements purify, balance, and activate the body's energy centers (or chakras, a Sanskrit word meaning wheel) to flow with Reiki energy effectively and efficiently.

In Japanese, the first degree, Reiki I, training is called *Shoden*, which means "the entrance." In this class, students are introduced to *Reiki Gokai* (the five Reiki precepts), principles of energy healing, and the history of Reiki. They are also introduced to hand positions for self-healing and beginning techniques for sharing Reiki with others in seated and lying-down positions. Depending on your teacher, you may also be taught techniques for learning how to clear disruptive energies in a space, a room, or a home and how to share Reiki with plants and animals as well. Understanding that Reiki requires a clear channel, this initial class focuses primarily on self-healing at the physical and etheric/energetic levels so that students can use Reiki to get clear and raise their personal vibration. You can easily see how the Reiki practitioner must first become a clear channel themselves in order to transmit this high-vibrational energy to others. Reiki I is an important part of this training and should not be rushed for any reason.

Classically, there is a twenty-one-day wait period between Reiki I and Reiki II training. This is to allow the energy to move through the full system and each of the seven main energy centers—allowing three days for each of the centers. Great cleansing, shift, and changes occur during this time.

It is advised that the student works with their Reiki energy every day to become familiar with its deeper wisdom. That is why this transformational period is so important. When the student is ready, without a sense of hurry, they may choose to move on to the next level of their training.

Reiki II training, known as *Okuden* in Japanese, translates to "the deep inside." At this level, students explore the Reiki symbols, which enhance various energetic qualities and focus in their Reiki practice. During this phase in their training, students learn to *send* Reiki over long distances to individuals who have provided informed consent to receive it. The Reiki II training offers deeper experiences in transmitting healing energies over time and space, dedicating substantial class time to practicing this important work. At this stage, there is a primary focus on achieving greater personal healing at the mental and emotional levels.

Traditionally, there is a one-year period of growth and transformation between Reiki II and Reiki III training.[19] This is not merely a passive waiting time but rather earnest work with the energies of the Divine presence, which becomes an ongoing healing practice. The Reiki student becomes a student of Reiki energy, dedicated to regular practice, learning from its strength, wisdom, and love. This period is designated as a movement of cyclical change, as the planet revolves around the sun, moving through each of the four seasons. Within each seasonal transformation, the Reiki practitioner is also transformed. When the student is ready, without a sense of hurry, they may choose to move on to the next level of their training.

In Japanese, Reiki III training is called *Shinpiden*, which means "mystery, secret teachings." This training is very spiritual and is undertaken only after at least a year-long committed period of deep personal growth with Reiki. At this point, Reiki III candidates will learn advanced healing techniques and work with the highest spiritual energies to assist others. The final attunement is considered a connection to the flame of enlightenment at the energy center at the top of the head, the crown chakra. In Western cultures, we will often call the Reiki III graduate a Reiki Master or Reiki Master Practitioner (RMP). In some schools, the Reiki III class provides training in how to attune others and to teach Reiki classes, as well. Some will separate this work into a distinct training course, with an additional attunement, and the graduate will then be conferred the title of Reiki Master Teacher (RMT).

Reiki classes are found in all areas of study, including colleges, universities, medical facilities, adult/community education programs, hospitals, and private practices worldwide. Certain training centers also offer children's classes for ages eight and over. Children's classes are usually level I only until the child reaches their late teens, when they may, more appropriately, move to the next level.

Practitioner Experience

Reiki practitioners may begin to treat others with Reiki at level II training and beyond. Although Reiki I practitioners are certainly welcome to share their Reiki energy, it is usually informally for their friends and family at this first stage. If you are seeking a session from a Reiki practitioner, you will want to know to what level they have received their training, remembering that the *professional* standard is Reiki III or Reiki Master. It is at this level that the practitioner can also join professional organizations that help support their practice and professional development.

Suppose you have friends or family who are offering to share their Reiki with you while they are still learning. This would be a terrific win-win opportunity, as you would both learn and investigate the beauty of energy healing together. Also, your feedback can be invaluable to one learning about their own Reiki energies. However, if you are paying for a professional session, it is best to ask a couple of questions or read about the practitioner's training and experience before you make the appointment.

In the United Kingdom, Reiki professionals are licensed and have a particular quality mark designated by the Complementary and Natural Healthcare Council (CNHC). This is a clear mark of their professional status. In the United States, at this time, Reiki is not federally licensed. It is left to the states to determine their governance of non-licensed alternative healthcare practitioners. Each state's laws and perspectives differ on this matter, and the rules frequently change. You will also find certain schools are "licensing" practitioners within their own organizations. This growing practice assures a certain uniformity of purpose, intention, and training, which aligns with the school's code of ethics and practice. However, this is not a state or federal license, and it varies widely.

It is up to you to exercise due diligence to find the practitioner that best suits you. Information about your professional practitioner's training and experience should be readily available on their website or whatever public interface they use. Suppose you do not find their training, credentials, and experience posted with their offerings. In that case, it is certainly appropriate to reach out (by email or phone) to ask about these matters before making an appointment. Suggested questions to ask are offered at the end of this chapter.

Commitment to the Work

For me, the length of time a Reiki practitioner has been in professional practice, or the number of sessions they have conducted on others, is far less important than their commitment to the work. A daily personal Reiki practice is imperative for the purity of the light they transmit. For this reason, even an overly scheduled practitioner who sees myriads of clients but does not work on themselves may not be as clear or as fully "connected" to the higher vibrations needed. This shines through in the purity of their light.

A professional practitioner is committed to self-healing work on a daily or near-daily basis. Through this regular practice, the channel maintains the clarity to transmit Reiki at high enough vibrational levels to assist others. When a practitioner is charging for their services, daily practice is a fundamental requirement for any committed light worker.

In choosing a practitioner, you may want to check in with your own intuitive sense. Meeting the basic requirement of daily (or near-daily) self-Reiki sessions, does this energetic purity resonate outward in their own energy field? Is their personal space charged with Divine presence? Is Reiki evident in their personal energetic flow—how they speak, how they carry themselves in the world, how they conduct their business, how they lead their lives? Do they appear to be living (or striving to live) the Reiki Principles, the Gokai, shared in Chapter 1, What Is Reiki?

Reiki, being Divine light, does not align with lower vibrational choices that move us out and away from our higher connection, like alcohol, non-prescription drugs, or anything that takes the conscious mind out of its center. Remaining centered in the light of Reiki generally means a commitment to higher vibrational actions and activities. For this reason, alcohol and drugs are never a part of Reiki and certainly should never be used during a session.

Of course, no one is perfect, and Reiki does not insist on perfection—thank goodness! However, Reiki can assist those on a path of self-improvement and soul growth, as its compassionate light helps them make higher-vibrational choices. That is the lightwork of Reiki.

Word of Mouth

Reiki practitioners often find their work to be their best advertisement. A happy and well-cared-for client will gladly share their experiences with others, letting friends and family know. Moreover, family and friends who witness the subtle (or profound) changes in someone who was previously struggling will want to know more about what they are doing that has positively impacted their lives. For that reason, clients will often share, recommend, and encourage those they care for to try Reiki for themselves.

The opposite is also true: a disgruntled client is more likely to post on social media platforms, sometimes anonymously, to share their unhappy experiences. We take it all with the proverbial grain of salt. Reiki has nothing to prove and will often not defend itself or argue with others' perceptions.

If you are seeking a qualified Reiki practitioner in your area, ask your friends, those who seek similar quality and experiences, if they know first-hand of someone you could see. Many practitioners work out of their homes, so you may not see storefronts or neon signs blinking, "Reiki!" There are many more practitioners in your area than you are probably aware of. For that reason, visiting your favorite search engine may also give you some direction if your friends and family are unfamiliar with Reiki practitioners. Hospitals, hospice programs, wellness centers, naturopathic physicians, palliative care programs, yoga studios, and meditation centers may have local Reiki practitioners they could recommend.

Some Reiki practitioners may offer low-cost or free events for the community—like Reiki circles, Reiki shares (described more fully in Chapter 2), discussion groups, and meditation workshops. These are terrific opportunities to meet the practitioner to get a sense of their style, approach, and overall energy. You may also be able to feel their Reiki in one of the Reiki shares or circles, so you can get a clearer sense of the practitioner's connection to Reiki. If time allows, you might be able to have a short discussion with them about their work. If it feels like a good fit for you, you might consider making an appointment for a private session.

Not every Reiki practitioner will be a good fit for everyone. That is okay. There is no need to discredit or complain about the practitioner. Just as Reiki practitioners aligning with the highest frequencies of unconditional love will never malign someone else's work, nothing positive comes from such energies, and lower vibrations can take hold within the practice of someone who is egotistically undercutting another practitioner's work. Instead, making every effort to rise above an unhealthy ego, the Reiki practitioner takes care of the soul of their practice by pouring light into both the practice and the business of Reiki.

Blessings to all.

For more information on choosing a professional Reiki practitioner, visit www.reikiintegrativemedicine.com.

Suggested Questions to Ask a Potential Reiki Therapist

What form(s) of Reiki do you practice?

There are close to a hundred forms of Reiki being practiced today around the world. The form of Reiki described most fully in this book is Usui Reiki. Medical Reiki is also referenced. Both of these are in alignment with and honor the Usui tradition of Reiki.

What is the highest level of training you have received?

Professional training is completed at the Third Degree/ Reiki III or Reiki Master level. Reiki Master Teacher training is a step beyond the Reiki Master (Practitioner) designation. Reiki II practitioners may also offer sessions even though they have not yet completed their professional training.

Did you receive your training with a teacher present for your attunements?

Professional organizations agree that asynchronous attunements, meaning without a teacher's presence ("sent" to the student without sharing time or space), are below the standards of traditional Reiki training. The teacher's presence is on par with in-person or online attunements as long as the student and the teacher share the experience live, synchronously, at the same time. This is so that the Reiki Master Teacher can hold space for the experience of attunement on the physical level.

How long have you been practicing Reiki professionally?
As mentioned, the length of time or the number of previous sessions given alone does not indicate the quality of the Reiki energy or the experience of it. However, there is much to learn about energy and healing. It is expected that the practitioner has been on a healing path for themselves to a significant degree *prior* to offering professional-level Reiki sessions to others or passing attunements.

How often do you use Reiki for yourself or give yourself Reiki treatments?
If the answer to this question is anything less than daily or near daily, this would most likely indicate that the practitioner is not living with the essence of Reiki. They may have different opinions about this, so it is good to have that discussion. Hear their understanding of Reiki and how it informs their lives. If it seems to align with your expectations, then trust your inner guidance. If it does not, then know that there are plenty of practitioners available.

Do you belong to any professional Reiki organizations?
There are numerous professional Reiki organizations available all around the world, from the local level through to the international level. Organizations support professional development and ongoing training for their members. A reputable practitioner who is committed to current research and professional development in their work will likely have a membership with one or more of the following

organizations or others like them, but this is certainly not a requirement. Here are a few examples of respected Reiki organizations:

- International Association of Reiki Professionals (IARP)
- International Center for Reiki Training (ICRT)
- The Reiki Alliance
- The Reiki Association
- Center for Reiki Research (CRR)

Seeking a Practitioner for a Clinical Setting

If you are seeking a practitioner who can come to the hospital, medical treatment center, or long-term care center, you may wish to ask the following questions:

- Do you provide Reiki sessions at hospitals/care centers?
- How long have you been working in medical/clinical Reiki settings?
- Are you trained to accompany a client into surgery? Do you know how to help me approach this topic with my surgeon?
- Do you offer distance Reiki during surgery or treatments?
- Are you trained in providing Reiki before, during, or after chemotherapy infusions?

In-depth questions for longer discussions might include:

- In your practice and experience, where does Reiki energy come from?
- Do you follow the Reiki Principles (Reiki Gokai)? What do they mean to you?
- What kind(s) of professional development activities do you participate in?

The Reiki Calling

For many, Reiki is a calling from the soul, urging us forward into the healing light of Divine service. It may start as a subtle curiosity, a wondering about energetic experiences that seem beyond the natural world's capacity. Then, perhaps synchronicities arise, and Reiki comes into your inner circle in uncanny ways—through mentions, discussions, or experiences. Reiki may begin to feel familiar beyond explanation.

Perhaps an inner impulse nudges you to learn more and explore the mystical experience of Reiki. You begin to lean in. First, a session or two. Then perhaps you realize that you *can* do this for yourself and those you love, and you begin to learn Reiki.

Training at the first level, Reiki I, is a class that is conducted over two to four days, somewhere between ten and fourteen hours in total. But the transformative effects of this training will last a lifetime. If you are so called to learn Reiki, you will have a deeper understanding of how energy works, how it is transferred, entangled, and released, and how it is best managed for the highest and best good for all. Great personal growth and healing can occur at the first Reiki training level.

I believe everyone would benefit from learning Reiki at this primary level of training. Reiki I is not about becoming a practitioner or starting a new business (although that can happen, too, with further training). Still, it is about understanding energetic flow and our interconnectedness beyond the physical body. It will heal the many aspects of your being: the physical, mental, emotional, and subtle energy bodies.

Reiki brings many blessings of infinite light and unconditional love into your life and your healing path. It assists
in clearing your energetic field, raising your frequency, and
growing your soul. May you continue to be blessed by the
call of Reiki.

CHAPTER 6

Frequently Asked Questions About Reiki

Throughout my years of practicing and teaching Reiki, certain questions come up fairly regularly. Here is a list of questions and brief answers that you or your loved ones may have about Reiki:

Is there a physical healing crisis associated with Reiki? That is, will I feel bad for a short amount of time after a session before I feel better?
No. Unlike other healing modalities, Reiki does not involve a healing crisis. There is no toxic or energetic "dump" into the bloodstream, nothing that the body has to filter out afterward, and no "die-off" that the physical body has to overcome after the session. At the end of the Reiki session, you should feel calm and clear; many even describe the sensation of feeling lighter after a session.

Some Reiki practitioners are also psychic mediums. Is that a part of Reiki?
No, Reiki practitioners are not involved in any form of psychic work, nor are they conducting "readings" during a Reiki session. Psychic medium work is another modality entirely and may even come from a different place than where Reiki energy originates. Reiki, in its purest form, is not psychic mediumship or psychic anything.

The Reiki practitioner who receives "messages" during sessions must be exceptionally discerning regarding the message's origin. The ego can convince someone that they are receiving from a higher vibrational plane than they are. This is where experience can be helpful. Also, part of the practitioner's Reiki training should have included the understanding that we are not there to diagnose, prescribe, or give direction based on the energy we experience.

Can Reiki heal (*fill in the blank*)?
Yes. *Reiki can heal anything and everything.* There are no limitations to Reiki. The limitations are always in our own thinking. However, remember that healing is different from a cure (see Chapter 3, Integrative Medicine, Medical Reiki, and Clinical Settings). Like the many layers of an onion, several layers of energetic imprints may surround any given issue for which you seek Reiki healing.

Reiki healing is always gentle and supportive and has a high vibration of light. It may take only one session to address the core cause of the disruptive energies or it may take much longer, your life's work, even. Simply allow Reiki to do its work, and know that healing is always taking place, leading you to the next step of your healing journey.

Will Reiki interfere with my medical treatments?
No. Reiki works well with all medical treatments and medications without contraindications. It is a gentle, non-invasive treatment that promotes the relaxation response so that the body, mind, and spirit can heal.

Your Reiki practitioner will never diagnose or prescribe treatments, and they will never suggest stopping any treatment prescribed by your doctor. Reiki is collaborative on all levels. Many hospitals and treatment programs offer Reiki as part of their integrative medicine or spiritual care programs.

Feel free to seek Reiki treatments to supplement the healing treatments prescribed by your doctor. As always, it is helpful and advised to let your physician know you are also using Reiki to assist on your healing journey.

How often should I receive Reiki treatments?
There is no standard answer to this question, as it entirely depends on the individual and the circumstance. I offer clients who are experiencing acute issues a distance asynchronous option, where they will receive distance Reiki support on three consecutive days to help them through a time of particular stress, pressure, or illness. This is a terrific supportive measure available with relative ease, and much can be shifted in this sort of process.

For others, in-person sessions are preferred. When someone is going through something rather intense, weekly sessions for a short period may be helpful. For others, monthly sessions give just the right amount of support for someone seeking personal growth, support, and self-care. Others, still, will seek Reiki seasonally and come in for a session with the change of the season to get clear and bring upliftment and healing light to their journey.

In Reiki, I generally suggest that the client ask for inner guidance as to when it is time to return. There may be times when you wish to receive Reiki more frequently and at other times less often. Allow yourself the freedom to go with the energetic flow when making your decisions. There are no minimum requirements and no maximum limits to the amount of Reiki you receive. Remember, if you choose to learn Reiki for yourself, even at the first level, you could give yourself treatments daily (or more often) if you so desire.

Is Reiki a cult or witchcraft?

No. And, no. I have heard both of these statements about Reiki, though, by those who know nothing about it. Reiki does not require anything from its clients or students, who are always free to decide when and if they wish to use its healing energies. Free will, as a gift of the Divine, is always honored in Reiki.

Witchcraft, or magic, does not honor the free will of the recipient, as the practitioners are setting their own intentions for self-serving outcomes. This is not the case with Reiki. Reiki practitioners do not create intentions that violate free will and the laws of Divine will. Reiki is always in service to Divine will, putting personal will aside for the highest good and the best outcome.

Is Reiki religious or anti-Christian?

Reiki has no religious-centric worldview. Like God, Reiki belongs to no religion and can work within all belief systems. The same could be said about prayer or meditation. Neither belong to any particular set of beliefs but are tools that allow individuals to connect more directly to their higher power. Reiki is not anti-any religious belief at all and is practiced by believers of all religions and those with no religious affiliation at all.

Should I see multiple Reiki practitioners for individual sessions during the same period?

Unless there is something that is not working with your current Reiki practitioner, it is probably best to see only one practitioner for the issue you are seeking assistance with. Seeing two or three different Reiki practitioners in private sessions throughout the week may not give you the results you are seeking. Remember that it is not the practitioner that is doing the healing; the practitioner is the delivery system. Unless you feel there is something out of alignment with your Reiki practitioner, you may want to allow the practitioner to deliver the energy. Trust in Reiki to do the work.

That being said, if you are not connected to your practitioner or you feel they are not connecting high enough to do the work well, feel free to find another practitioner. No explanations are needed.

Do you have a question about Reiki that wasn't covered here?

Ask your question at www.reikiintegrativemedicine.com.

References

1. Archangel Gabriel to M. Lori Torok (2014). Over the years, my inner guidance and higher communication with spiritual messengers have developed through my work with Reiki. This quote was given to me by Archangel Gabriel in answer to my question about how best to describe the flow of energy during a Reiki transmission.

2. This is attributed to Heraclitus, (535–475 BCE) as found in Plato's Cratylus (402a).

3. This data is from a 2007 study by Dr. Ann Vitale found at UCLAhealth. org. The numbers are considerably higher now.

4. Sheldon Marc Feldman, M.D., FACS. "Medical Reiki Works meeting for CMRMs to Learn How Raven's Legacy Continues," Medical Reiki Works, New York. January 25, 2024.

5. U.S. Department of Veteran Affairs. "Passport to Whole Health." Available at https://www.va.gov/wholehealthlibrary/passport/chapter-17. asp

6. U.S. Department of Veteran Affairs. "Passport to Whole Health." Available at https://www.va.gov/WHOLEHEALTHLIBRARY/passport/ index.asp

7. Redd, D., Zeng-Treitler, Q., Brandt, C., Shao, Y., Goulet, J. (2020) "Using explainable deep learning and logistic regression to evaluate complementary and integrative health treatments in patients with musculoskeletal disorders," Proceedings of the 53rd Hawaii International Conference on System Sciences, 2020. Manoa Community, Hawaii: Scholar Space, 1–9.

8. National Center for Health Statistics. (2012) "2012 National Health Interview Survey." Available at: https://www.cdc.gov/nchs/index.htm

9. Kluge, H. (2023) Statement by Dr Hans Henri P. Kluge, WHO Regional

Director for Europe, at the conclusion of the WHO Traditional Medicine Global Summit in Gandhinagar, India, 18 August. Available at https://www.who.int/europe/news

10. Dyer, N., Baldwin, A., Rand, W. (2019) "A large-scale effectiveness trial of Reiki for physical and psychological health," *The Journal of Alternative and Complementary Medicine*, 25(12), pp 1156–1162. Available at https://www.liebertpub.com/doi/abs/10.1089/acm.2019.0022

11. Díaz-Rodríguez, L., Arroyo-Morales, M., Fernández-de-las-Peñas, C., García-Lafuente, F., García-Royo, C., Tomás-Rojas, I. (2011) "Immediate effects of Reiki on Heart Rate Variability, cortisol levels, and body temperature in health care professionals with burnout," *Biological Research for Nursing*, 13(4), pp 376–382. doi:10.1177/1099800410389166. Used by licensed permission.

12. Rafaq, F., Haider, S., Sheikh, F. (2022) "The effects of Reiki treatment on mental health professionals who are at risk of burnout," *Int. j. adv. multidisc. res. stud.*, 2(4), pp 519–522. Available at https://www.academia.edu/84213067/The_effects_of_Reiki_treatment_on_mental_health_professionals_who_are_at_risk_of_burnout?f_ri=276837

13. Kundu, A. (2013) "Reiki training for caregivers of hospitalized pediatric patients: A pilot program," *Complementary Therapies in Clinical Practice: Elsevier*, February. Used by licensed permission.

14. Yüce, U. and Taşcı, S. (2021) "Effect of Reiki on the stress level of caregivers of patients with cancer: Qualitative and single-blind randomized controlled trial," *Complementary Therapies in Medicine*, 58, 102708, ISSN 0965-2299. Available at https://doi.org/10.1016/j.ctim.2021.102708; https://www.sciencedirect.com/science/article/pii/S0965229921000492. Used under Creative Commons and licensed permission.

15. Utli, H., Dinç, M., Utli, A. (2023) "The effect of acupressure or Reiki interventions on the levels of pain and fatigue of cancer patients receiving palliative care: A randomized controlled study," *EXPLORE*, 19(1), pp 91–99. ISSN 1550-8307. Available at: https://doi.org/10.1016/j.explore.2022.11.007. Used with licensed permission.

16. Şişman, H. and Arslan, S. (2023) "The effect of Reiki on anxiety, fear, pain, and oxygen saturation in abdominal surgery patients: A randomized controlled trial," *EXPLORE*, 19(4), pp 578–586, ISSN 1550-8307. Available at https://doi.org/10.1016/j.explore.2022.11.005. Used with licensed permission.

17. Dyer, N., Rodgers-Melnick, S., Fink, K., Rao, S., Surdam, J., Dusek, J. (2025) "Evaluation of a Reiki Volunteer Program within Two Cancer Infusion Centers," *Journal of Pain and Symptom Management*, vol 69: 3, pp e211 – e219. Available at: https://www.jpsmjournal.com/article/S0885-3924(24)01132-1/abstract.

18. Different traditions and schools may vary regarding the number of attunements given at each Reiki degree.

19. Some traditions and schools have shortened this period to six months.

Appendix

Below are examples of intake paperwork for a professional Reiki session.

Name: (Please Print)_____

Phone (home): _____

Cell phone: _____

Address: _____

_____

City, State, Zip:_____

Age:_____

Email: _____

Date of Birth: _____

Emergency Contact (name & phone): _____

_____

_____

Reason for today's visit, in general (choose all that apply):

___physical healing   ___stress/anxiety

___depression   ___emotional support

___spiritual support   ___seeking clarity

___disruptive sleep   ___psychic/energetic attack

___curiosity   ___ other: _____

_____

Are you currently under the care of a physician for your condition(s)?

___ Yes ___ No

If yes, the physician's name: _____

_____

Have you ever had a Reiki session before? ___Yes ___No

If yes, when was your last session? _____

Number of previous sessions _____

How did you hear about us? _____

_____

Are you comfortable with the use of essential oils during your session? ___Yes ___No

Do you prefer/request a hands-off (no touch) session?

___Yes ___No

Females: Are you pregnant? ___Yes ___No ___Possibly

Client Informed Consent

I understand the following:
- Reiki is a simple, gentle, hands-on energy technique used for stress reduction and relaxation.
- I understand that the body has the ability to heal itself, and complete relaxation is often beneficial.
- Reiki gently promotes relaxation so that the body can heal itself.
- I can choose a hands-off (no touch) session at any time if I prefer.

- Reiki practitioners do not diagnose conditions, perform medical treatment, prescribe medicine, or interfere with the treatment of a licensed medical professional.
- Reiki does not replace medical care. It is recommended that I see a licensed physician or licensed healthcare professional for any physical or psychological ailment I may have.
- I understand that Reiki can complement any medical or psychological care I may be receiving.
- Although most will experience relief from just one Reiki session, I acknowledge that long-term imbalances in the body sometimes require multiple sessions to facilitate the level of relaxation needed by the body to heal itself. The number and frequency of sessions is always up to the client.

_____

Signature

_____

Date

Privacy Statement

No specific/identifying information about any client will be discussed or shared with *any* third party without the client's written consent (or parent/guardian if the client is under 18) *unless* the client presents a concern as a harm to him/herself or others. I acknowledge this privacy agreement with my signature below:

Client Signature: _____

Eloia Healing Arts' Signature:_____

Practitioner Credentials and Disclosure

California Senate Bill 577 requires alternative healthcare practitioners to provide the following information to their clients:

- *The State of California does not license Reiki Therapists, Sound Healing Therapists, End-of-Life Doulas, or Bach Flower Essence consultants; these modalities are NOT intended to replace traditional Western medical or mental health treatments.*
- *Your practitioner, M. Lori Torok, holds a **Bachelor of Arts** degree from **Niagara University (1990)** and a **Master of Arts** degree from the **State University of New York at Brockport (1992)**, where she trained and taught in dance, movement techniques, and somatic modalities.*
- *M. Lori Torok has earned the third degree/Reiki Master level under three distinct lineages:*
  - *Usui Reiki Healing Method, Reiki Master Teacher (2013)*
  - *Karuna Reiki Master Teacher (2017)*
  - *Certified Medical Reiki Master (2022)*
- *Your practitioner, M. Lori Torok, has completed certificated training in the following programs:*
  - *Bach Flower Essence Practitioner at the Bach Centre in England*
    - *BFRP – Bach Foundation Registered Practitioner*
    - *Practitioner Number: USA-2020-0428K*
  - *Sound Healing Practitioner - Ascending Sounds (2014)*
  - *Allergy Desensitization – Blossom Health & Wellness (2011)*

- ◆ *Oncology Reiki – Huntington Beach Reiki (2014)*
- ◆ *End-of-Life Doula Certificate – University of Vermont, Osher Center for Integrative Health (2024)*
- *M. Lori Torok has been in private practice since 2013 and opened **Eloia Healing Arts | Temecula Reiki & Sound Therapy** in 2014.*
- *M. Lori Torok is an ordained minister (2011) with Universal Life Church and is credentialed to legally officiate sacred ceremonies, such as weddings, baptisms, memorials/celebrations of life, and any other sacred rites you may need on your journey.*
- *Professional memberships & affiliations in good standing:*
  - ◆ *International Center for Reiki Training (ICRT)*
  - ◆ *Center for Reiki Research (CRR)*
  - ◆ *Sound Healing Association (SHA)*
  - ◆ *Bach Foundation International Register of Practitioners (BRFP)*
  - ◆ *Raven Keyes Medical Reiki International (RKMRI)*
  - ◆ *The Reiki Association (TRA/UK)*
  - ◆ *International Association of Reiki Practitioners (IARP)*

My signature below indicates that I have received and read the information provided about this practitioner's training and qualifications per CA-SB577.

_____

Signature

_____

Date

Bibliography

Alfred, J. (2006) *Our Invisible Bodies: Scientific Evidence for Subtle Bodies*. Indiana: Trafford Publishing.

America Board of Physician Specialties. "Integrative Medicine Defined." Available at https://www.abpsus.org/integrative-medicine-defined/.

Baldwin, A. (2021) *Reiki in Clinical Practice: A Science-Based Guide*. UK: Handspring Publishing.

Becker, R. & Selden, G. (1998) *The Body Electric: Electromagnetism and the Foundation of Life*. New York: William Morrow.

Brennan, B. (1988) *Hands of Light: A Guide to Healing Through the Human Energy Field*. New York: Bantam.

Center for Integrative Medicine. "What is Integrative Medicine?" Available at https://integrativemedicine.arizona.edu/health_hub/awcimagazine/what_is_integrative_medicine.html, accessed 5/30/2024.

Childre, D. and Martin, H. (2000). *The Heartmath Solution*. San Francisco: HarperOne.

Díaz-Rodríguez, L., Arroyo-Morales, M., Fernández-de-las-Peñas, C., García-Lafuente, F., García-Royo, C., Tomás-Rojas, I. (2011) "Immediate effects of Reiki on Heart Rate Variability, cortisol levels, and body temperature in health care professionals with burnout," *Biological Research for Nursing*, 13(4), pp 376–382. Available at doi:10.1177/1099800410389166

Doi, H. (2014) *A Modern Reiki Method for Healing.* Michigan: Vision Publications.

Dyer, N., Baldwin, A., & Rand, W. (2019) "A large-scale effectiveness trial of Reiki for physical and psychological health," *The Journal of Alternative and Complementary Medicine,* 25(12), pp 1156–1162. Available at https://www.liebertpub.com/doi/abs/10.1089/acm.2019.0022

Dyer, N., Rodgers-Melnick, S., Fink, K., Rao, S., Surdam, J., Dusek, J. (2025) "Evaluation of a Reiki Volunteer Program within Two Cancer Infusion Centers," *Journal of Pain and Symptom Management,* vol 69: 3, pp e211 – e219. Available at: https://www.jpsmjournal.com/article/S0885-3924(24)01132-1/abstract.

Feldman, S. (2024) "Medical Reiki Works Meeting for CMRMs to Learn How Raven's Legacy Continues," Medical Reiki Works, New York. January 25.

Gerber, R. (2001) *Vibrational Medicine.* Vermont: Bear & Company.

Gordon, Richard. (2006) *Quantum Touch: The Power to Heal.* California: North Atlantic Books.

Hamilton, D. (2021) *Why Woo-Woo Works: The Surprising Science Behind Meditation, Reiki, Crystals, and Other Alternative Practices.* California: Hay House.

International Association of Reiki Professionals. Available at: https://www.IARP.org

The International Center for Reiki Training. Available at https://www.reiki.org

Keyes, R. (2012) *The Healing Power of Reiki*. Minnesota: Llewelyn Publications.

_____ (2017) *The Healing Light of Angels*. Minnesota: Llewellyn Publications.

_____ (2021) *Medical Reiki*. Minnesota: Llewellyn Publications.

Kluge, H. (2023). Statement by Dr Hans Henri P. Kluge, WHO Regional Director for Europe, the conclusion of the WHO Traditional Medicine Global Summit in Gandhinagar, India, August 18. Available at https://www.who.int/europe/news

Kundu, A. (2013) "Reiki training for caregivers of hospitalized pediatric patients: A pilot program," *Complementary Therapies in Clinical Practice*: Elsevier, February.

Leskowitz, E. (2024) *The Mystery of Life Energy*. Vermont: Bear & Co.

Lipton, B. (2005) *The Biology of Belief: Unleashing the Power of Consciousness, Matter, and Miracles*. New York: Hay House.

Lübeck, W. and Petter, F. (2003) *Reiki: Best Practices*. Wisconsin: Lotus Press.

McKusick, E. (2014) *Tuning the Human Biofield: Healing with Vibrational Sound Therapy*. Rochester, Vermont: Healing Arts Press.

Miller, J. (2006) *Reiki's Birthplace: A Guide to Kurama Mountain*. Arizona: Infinite Light Healing Studies Center.

Myss, C. (1997) *Anatomy of the Spirit: The Seven Stages of Power and Healing.* New York: Harmony.

National Center for Complementary and Integrative Health. "Reiki." Available at https://www.nccih.nih.gov/health/reiki.

National Center for Health Statistics. "2012 National Health Interview Survey." Available at: https://www.cdc.gov/nchs/index.htm

Passport to Whole Health. "Energy Medicine: Biofield Therapies." Available at: https://www.va.gov/whole-healthlibrary/passport/chapter-17.asp.

Quest, P. (2011) *The Reiki Manual.* New York: Tarcher/Penguin.

Rafaq, F., Haider, S., Sheikh, F. (2022) "The effects of Reiki treatment on mental health professionals who are at risk of burnout," *Int. j. adv. multidisc. res. stud,* 2(4), pp 519–522. Available at https://www.academia.edu/84213067/The_effects_of_Reiki_treatment_on_mental_health_professionals_who_are_at_risk_of_burnout?f_ri=276837

Rand, W. (2014) *An Evidence Based History of Reiki.* Michigan: International Center for Reiki Training.

Raven Keyes Medical Reiki International. Available at: https://www.ravenkeyesmedicalreiki.com/

Redd, D., Zeng-Treitler, Q., Brandt, C., Shao, Y., Goulet, J. (2020) "Using explainable deep learning and logistic regression to evaluate complementary and integrative health treatments in patients with musculoskeletal disorders," Proceedings of the 53rd Hawaii International Conference on System Sciences. Manoa Community, Hawaii: Scholar Space, 1–9.

The Reiki Association. Available at https://www.reikiassociation.net

San Diego Reiki Corps. Available at https://www.sandiegoreikicorps.org/

Şişman, H. and Arslan, S. (2023) "The effect of Reiki on anxiety, fear, pain, and oxygen saturation in abdominal surgery patients: A randomized controlled trial," *EXPLORE,* 19(4), pp 578–586, ISSN 1550-8307. Available at https://doi.org/10.1016/j.explore.2022.11.005.

Stein, D. (1995) *Essential Reiki: A Complete Guide to an Ancient Healing Art.* New York: Crossing Press.

Torok, M. (2023) *Forgiveness: Journey to a Clear Place.* California: Eighth Ray Publishing.

UK Reiki Federation. Available at https://www.reikifed.co.uk

Usui, M. and Arjava Petter, F. (2011) *The Original Reiki Handbook of Dr. Mikao Usui.* Twin Lakes, Wisconsin: Lotus Press.

Utli, H., Dinç, M., Utli, A. (2023) "The effect of acupressure or Reiki interventions on the levels of pain and fatigue of cancer patients receiving palliative care: A randomized controlled study," *EXPLORE,* 19(1), pp 91–99. ISSN 1550-8307. Available at: https://doi.org/10.1016/j.explore.2022.11.007

Vitale, A. (2007) "An Integrative Review of Reiki Touch Therapy Research." Available at UCLAhealth.org.

Yamaguchi, T. (2007) *Light on the Origins of Reiki*. Twin Lakes, Wisconsin: Lotus Press.

Yüce, U. and Taşcı, S. (2021) "Effect of Reiki on the stress level of caregivers of patients with cancer: Qualitative and single-blind randomized controlled trial, *Complementary Therapies in Medicine*, 58, 102708, ISSN 0965-2299. Available at https://doi.org/10.1016/j.ctim.2021.102708.

Acknowledgments

I wish to acknowledge the dozens of clients who have come through my doors at Eloia Healing Arts over the past fourteen years, asking me for the book to help them learn more about Reiki. And I want to give a nod to the dozens of students who have asked for the book they could give to their families and friends that will help explain what Reiki is— and assure them of what it isn't. And I want to thank the medical professionals, therapists, first responders, soldiers, and veterans who have come into my biofield to ask where they can read more about Reiki because their experience was so profound that they just don't know how to process this work. Although there are other excellent resources tailored to different audiences, I knew I needed to answer the call of those who wanted to learn more *about* Reiki without learning how to *do* Reiki. This book was born out of necessity, and it wouldn't have come into existence without you. Thank you for asking.

I thank the heavens that I was led to my teacher, Raven Keyes. I am blessed to have shared time and space, ever so briefly, while she was in embodiment. Thank you, dear Raven—blessings to your soul. Thank you, Medical Reiki Works, Raven Keyes Medical Reiki International, and Dr. Sheldon Marc Feldman, for continuing Raven's work in research and education.

I want to thank Dr. Sanjay Muttreja for his open-hearted generosity in giving me a place to speak about Reiki at the Southwest Healthcare System symposium. His continued support of Reiki and how it can assist in caring for the caregiver gave me the solid ground needed to create this work.

Thank you to those who have supported the development of this book and those whose energetic imprints are felt throughout its pages. Thank you to my superb editor, Sandy Draper. Thank you, Jennifer Federico Stimson, for the design and one more reason to love Canada! Thank you Sandy Blood for your index wizardry. Big Reiki hugs to Anne Watson, Erica Russo, Mary-Scott Carpenter, Manpreet Rai, Heather Norlund, Kimberly Sherwood, Micaela Larson, Jennifer Voss, Michelle Jones, and many others.

I want to acknowledge the Center for Reiki Research, the International Center for Reiki Training. I appreciate all that you do in support of Reiki and its practitioners.

I want to acknowledge the support I continually receive from the Hay House Writer's Community and the excellent resources they provide.

Finally, I wish to thank my family—old and new—for the many ways family has meaning in my life. I am amazed and blessed by our shared journey and am grateful to walk this path with each of you. Steve, thank you for your love and support as we travel the labyrinth together. Zoë Leana, you are an inspiration and the light of my life. Thank you.

About the Author

M. Lori Torok is an integrative healthcare practitioner and owner of Eloia Healing Arts at Temecula Reiki & Sound Therapy, a thriving practice in Southern California. She is dedicated to assisting individuals on their path of health and wellness. Since opening her private practice in 2014, Lori has helped thousands of clients with Reiki and sound healing techniques, leading to relaxation, integrative wellness, and healing outcomes in body, mind, and spirit.

Lori is a Certified Medical Reiki Master (CMRM) through Raven Keyes Medical Reiki International, which supports the advanced training of Reiki practitioners in Energy Medicine, Integrative Medicine, and Complementary Medicine. She is a certified Reiki Master Teacher (RMT) in the Usui tradition, a Holy Fire® Karuna Reiki® Master, and has earned certificates in Oncology Reiki, Shamanic Reiki, Sound Healing, and an End-of-Life Doula Professional Certificate from the University of Vermont–Osher Center for Integrative Health.

She holds a Bachelor's degree (BA) from Niagara University and a Master of Arts (MA) from the State University of New York at Brockport. She studied flower essence therapy at the Bach Centre in Wallingford, England, and she is on the international registry of the Bach Foundation of Registered Practitioners (BFRP).

M. Lori Torok is the author of *FORGIVENESS: Journey to a Clear Place* (2023), an Amazon #1 best seller in Mysticism & Spirituality. Lori has published multiple articles in the international *Reiki News Magazine* and online publications such as *New Earth Consciousness* and *Know Thyself; Heal Thyself.*

Lori speaks about Reiki in integrative medicine, provides training for medical personnel, presents at corporate events, and facilitates engaging workshops.

More information is found at the following sites:

www.reikiintegrativemedicine.com

www.eloiahealingarts.com

www.mloritorok.com

Also Available from M. Lori Torok

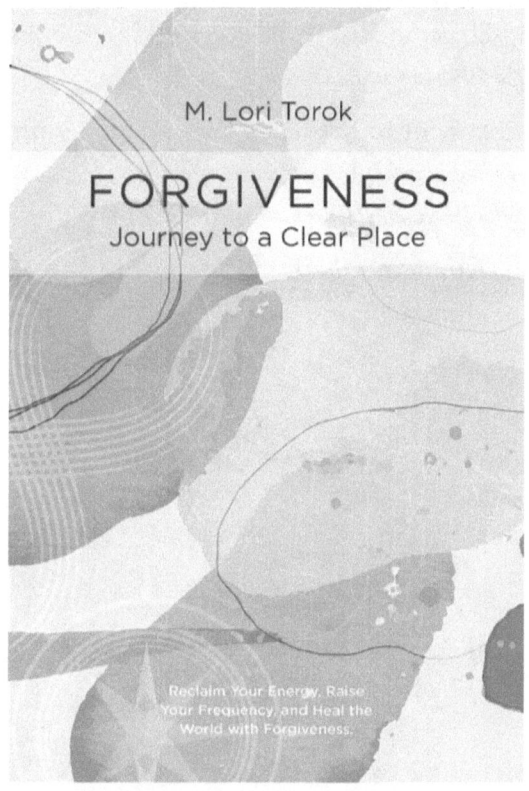

FORGIVENESS is energy medicine! Praise for Forgiveness: Journey to a Clear Place

"Torok approaches the hard task of forgiveness from several angles...and her gentle compassion shines through."

"Torok offers a robust and spiritual approach to letting go of resentments."

Kirkus Reviews

"A wonderful guide for anyone struggling to forgive themselves and others."

"Torok does such an excellent job discussing all facets of spiritual healing. Readers with a deep relationship with spirit and metaphysics will love *Forgiveness*."

Voted #20 on the list of Best Book Club Books 2023.

The Independent Book Review

"…a testament to her hard work and determination to heal the world through forgiveness."

Anna Pettit, HayHouseInc/Hay House Writer's Community

#1 on Amazon's New Releases in Mysticism & Spirituality, June 2023.

Index

E

effects (of Reiki treatments), 55–57, 58–61
empowerments. *See* attunements
energy, Reiki, 25, 30–31, 32
energy centers (chakras), 46, 93, 95
entrainment, 32
evidence-based studies, 69, 84–89

F

family dynamics, 35
Feldman, Sheldon M., 67–68, 77
five precepts *(Reiki Gokai)*, 27–30, 93
free will, 27, 43, 52, 108

G

gratitude, 29
grief, 79–80

H

Hartford Hospital, 73–74
healing crisis, 58, 105
healing *vs.* curing, 31–33, 106
healthcare
    alternative *vs.* integrative, 72
    patient-driven, 72–73
Healthcare Savings Plan (HSP), 69
health insurance, 68–70
heart rate variability (HRV), 56, 85
heart resonance, 32
hospice, 37, 79–80
hospitals

questions to ask, 100–102
seeing different practitioners, 53, 108–109
word of mouth recommendations, 98–100
psychic mediumship, 105–106
PTSD (post-traumatic stress disorder), xxii, 36

Q

qi, 25, 54, 55

R

Raven Keyes Medical Reiki International (RKMRI), 77
recuperation, 78
reflexology, 38–39
Reiki
described, 25–27
as bridge of light, 39–40
as a calling, xviii, 103–104
as Divine light, 31, 33, 61, 78, 98
effects of, 55–57, 58–61
five precepts, 27–30, 93
forms of, 25, 91, 100
life force energy, 25, 30–31, 32
as love, 32
massage *vs.*, 38–39, 44
origin of, 30–31
people who benefit from, 34–38, 57
professional organizations, 101–102
relaxation and, 79
souls and, 39–40
as supplement to medical treatments, 33–34, 36–37,
        68, 106–107

V

VA (US Dept. of Veterans Affairs), xx, 36, 70–72
vibration, law of, 29, 60
vibrational frequency, 32, 34
virtual sessions, 48–50

W

Weil, Andrew, 65
Whole Health program, 70–72
word of mouth recommendations, 98–100
working in service, 29–30
worry, 28–29

www.ingramcontent.com/pod-product-compliance
Lightning Source LLC
Chambersburg PA
CBHW021113130626
46554CB00002B/669